THE PREMATURE
LABOR HANDBOOK

THE PREMATURE LABOR HANDBOOK

Successfully Sustaining Your High-Risk Pregnancy

Patricia Anne Robertson, M.D.
Peggy Henning Berlin, Ph.D.

Drawings by Cindy P. Gates
with photographs by Hella Hammid

Doubleday & Company, Inc., Garden City, New York   1986

"Slow-Paced Breathing" by Susan Hilbers is reprinted with permission from *Genesis*, the bimonthly magazine on pregnancy and childbirth, published by ASPO/Lamaze, 1840 Wilson Boulevard, Suite 204, Arlington, VA 22201.

Excerpt from *Tao Te Ching*, by Lao Tsu, translated by Gia-fu Feng and Jane English, copyright © 1972 by Gia-fu Feng and Jane English, is reprinted by permission of Alfred A. Knopf, Inc.

Library of Congress Cataloging in Publication Data
Robertson, Patricia Anne.
    Premature labor handbook
    Bibliography: p. 205
    Includes index.
    1. Labor, Premature. 2. Labor, Premature—Psychological aspects. 3. Infants (Premature)—Hospital care. 4. Infants (Premature)—Care and hygiene. 5. Postnatal care. I. Berlin, Peggy Henning. II. Title.
RG649.R63 1986   618.5   85-10170
ISBN: 0-385-19923-6
ISBN: 0-385-19924-4(pbk)

ACKNOWLEDGMENTS

This book represents the loving and dedicated concern of a number of people who have experienced, from several different vantage points, premature labor and incompetent cervix. The book might not have been written were it not for the attitudes and treatment practices of a unique group of obstetric practitioners, Women's Medical Group of Santa Monica (Karen Blanchard, M.D., James Gordon, M.D., Marki Knox, M.D., Patricia Robertson, M.D., and Jacqueline Snow, M.N., N.P.). These clinicians embody the commitment to informed and collaborative patient care that inspired our writings. As a result of their conservative medical practice when preterm cervical change occurs, and their availability to support patients through anxious months of bedrest, their success in preventing premature birth has been remarkably high. We gratefully acknowledge the financial support of the Women's Health Research Foundation that has permitted the research and writing of this book. We wish especially to thank: Jacqueline Snow, M.N., N.P., for her help in creating the exercise chapter; Jeffrey Wasson, M.D., for his assistance from a pediatrician's viewpoint with the chapter regarding premature babies; and James Gordon, M.D., and Marie Herron, R.N., for their critical review of the entire manuscript.

The conceptual framework, tone, and organization of this book were fashioned from the principles and philosophy of MAXXIS, Inc., an organization of psychologists and training specialists offering programs to maximize personal effectiveness. It is their vision of the human capacity to create challenge from adversity and meaning from doubt that inspired at least one of us through premature labor and catalyzed the underlying message of this book. Their emphasis on five components—stress utilization, relationships, time, physical health, and personal creativity (including visualization)—clearly provided the outline for much of our presentation approach. We wish to thank particularly Jan Berlin, Ph.D., for his editorial infusion of inspiration, and Michele Thompson for her suggestions regarding the design of the book for training purposes. We extend special thanks to Deborah Brown for word processing.

For this book to become a reality in the public eye required some interesting turns of events and generous acts of belief. We would like to thank Sara Davidson for her interest and constant support for our vision of publishing this book. We are especially grateful to Kate Medina and Jennifer Brehl, not only for their editorial wisdom and skill, but also for their belief in the importance of early detection and prevention of high-risk pregnancies. Their commitment to public education and personal participation in medical treatment has helped to mold this book. We especially thank them for their flexibility in making it so.

Finally, of course, we acknowledge and celebrate those from whom came the observations, advice, and inspiration—premature labor patients and their families. We have been continually impressed with the integrity with which many families meet the demands of this challenging time. We only hope we can convey to others the spirit and resolve that enabled them to "hold on." In attempting to do so, we dedicate this book to our children, Geoffrey and Kate, and to the many other children who indeed begin to be their parents' teachers, even in the womb.

CONTENTS

6. THE HOSPITAL EXPERIENCE   110
By Mary Sue Ulven, R.N., and Patricia Robertson, M.D.

7. PRETERM DELIVERY AND THE PREMATURE BABY   121

LIST OF FIGURES

FIGURE

INTRODUCTION

Experiencing complications during pregnancy usually comes as a surprise. You may have heard from friends or colleagues about someone having to go to bed for the duration of her pregnancy—but how could this ever happen to *you?* You may have done everything "right": given up your usual morning coffee in early pregnancy, willingly or unwillingly gone to special prenatal exercise classes, attended all of your scheduled prenatal visits. Why should premature labor happen to you?

In the majority of cases, the causes of premature labor or an incompetent cervix are not known. About 8 to 10 percent of all pregnancies are affected by these conditions. If you have been diagnosed with one of these conditions, your pregnancy plans will have to change. The important thing to remember is that you are lucky in one respect: your practitioner has made a diagnosis early enough so that a miscarriage or premature birth can hopefully be prevented. Something can be done about it.

This book is written for you and for your partner and family, so that all of you can understand the importance of prolonging your pregnancy to the point when your baby can safely be born. However, with that process comes the unexpected: bedrest, possibly medication, and occasionally the birth of a premature baby. The change in your world, be it as a career woman or a homemaker, is profound. You are being challenged to nurture your baby in a special way, to insure the baby's maximal health. This challenge can be met with passive acceptance and resentment, or with enthusiasm and knowledge.

The chapters in this book contain information not only on the medical aspects of premature labor, incompetent cervix, and premature delivery, but also on how to cope with the stress of this new challenge and how to meet this challenge constructively. We hope the book will help you in many ways during these difficult weeks or months.

The extended time in the womb that you will be able to accomplish for your unborn child is tremendously important in giving your child an optimal start in life. We wish you the best of luck with your journey!

Patty Robertson, M.D.
Peggy Berlin, Ph.D.

THE PREMATURE
LABOR HANDBOOK

1

THE MEDICAL ASPECTS OF PREMATURE LABOR AND WEAKENED OR "INCOMPETENT" CERVIX

PREMATURE LABOR

I first thought that the baby was being especially active after dinner. Then all night I had what I thought were gas pains three or four times an hour. The next morning there were definite tightenings of my uterus and I saw my obstetrician. My cervix was two centimeters dilated and 80 percent effaced, and I was only thirty weeks pregnant! On the monitor, to my surprise, I was having contractions every three minutes. I was immediately admitted to the hospital, and after two days of medication and bedrest, the contractions were under control. What a scare!

> A mother who delivered a
> healthy baby at term,
> after eight weeks of bedrest.

Approximately 6 percent to 8 percent of all pregnant women develop the condition of premature or preterm labor. Preterm labor is defined as uterine contractions causing cervical change before thirty-seven weeks of pregnancy are completed (the normal length of pregnancy is forty weeks). If the preterm labor is not treated, 70 percent to 80 percent of these pregnancies will end prematurely, before the newborn infant is optimally ready to adapt to an environment outside the womb. Problems of premature newborn infants include immature lungs, often requiring the assistance of a breathing machine (respirator); life-threatening infections; and problems with bowel function. Often these premature infants require months of hospitalization in an Intensive Care Nursery. There is concern not only about short-term survival from immediate medical problems, but about long-term neurological outcome (e.g., an episode of intracranial bleeding in a premature newborn can cause permanent brain damage). About 75 percent of newborn problems occur in relation to premature birth. You can see, therefore, how essential it is to prevent a premature birth.

In the 1980s great strides have taken place in the detection and treatment of preterm labor, significantly reducing the incidence of preterm births. However, the treatment of preterm labor involves a great commitment from the pregnant woman, her partner, and her family. It means that an active life suddenly becomes one of bedrest. Often medication is necessary for the treatment of premature labor. A whole new sphere of medical terminology, hospitals, and medications envelop both the pregnant woman in preterm labor and her partner. Time is of the essence, and often a detailed explanation of the ongoing events and options is not available. The purpose of this chapter is to acquaint you with the concept of preterm labor, and to explain the different regimens available for its treatment.

THE DEFINITION OF PRETERM LABOR

Most women have some contractions of the uterus (uterine "tightenings") during pregnancy, apart from those that occur in the labor process. These occasional uterine contractions are known as "Braxton-Hicks." The difference between Braxton-Hicks contractions and those of premature labor is that the Braxton-Hicks contractions do not alter the cervix—that is, they do not dilate it or thin it out.

Preterm labor is the occurrence of frequent uterine contractions in the presence of progressive cervical change prior to thirty-seven weeks of pregnancy. For instance, one woman may have contractions throughout her pregnancy with no effect on the cervix. The cervix of another pregnant woman, however, who has the same quantity and quality of contractions for only a day, may become dilated and effaced, predisposing her to a premature birth. The first of these women is not in premature labor; the second is. Usually the contractions need to be ten to fifteen minutes apart (or less) on a regular basis to change the cervix.

THE ANATOMY OF PRETERM LABOR

The uterus is an incredible organ. In its nonpregnant state it is the size of a small pear. At term (nine months of pregnancy or gestation) it has expanded to encompass a seven- to eight-lb. baby, a placenta, and amniotic fluid.

The top portion of the uterus is the fundus, the lower portion is the lower uterine segment, while the bottom part of the uterus is the cervix, which protrudes into the vagina (see Figure 1). The cervix in a nonpregnant state is approximately four centimeters long (1 inch = 2.5 cm). This length is measured from the internal os (opening) to the external os. The cervix in its nonpregnant state is firm in texture and is closed tightly at the internal os. The cervix assumes various angles in the vagina, depending on the position of the uterus. Once the uterus contains a pregnancy, the cervix softens, but should not significantly thin out (efface) or dilate until the last month of pregnancy.

Five different parameters are used in evaluating the cervix in pregnancy: dilation, effacement, texture, angle, and the position of the fetus in relationship to the pelvis and cervix.

The *dilation* of the cervix is the most obvious change during preterm labor. A cervix that is three to four centimeters (cm) open instead of tightly closed at seven months of pregnancy often indicates that delivery is imminent. Premature rupture of the amniotic sac (membranes) surrounding the fetus may also easily occur once the cervix is prematurely dilated, which can also represent an imminent delivery. Once a significant amount of cervical dilation has occurred, preterm labor is much more difficult to treat than if only cervical effacement has occurred.

Cervical *effacement,* or thinning and shortening of the cervix, usually takes place before dilation of the cervix. The effacement can occur in varying degrees. A cervix in pregnancy that is not thinned out at all is about three to four cm long, and is termed 0 percent effaced. A cervix that is completely thinned out in pregnancy is termed 100 percent effaced. The next step (since there is no more cervix to efface) would be dilation. Between these two extremes of effacement, there are other possibilities. Most of them are described in terms of percent of effacement in degrees of ten, e.g., 50 percent effaced, 80 percent effaced, and so forth. However, some clinicians describe cervical effacement in terms of length, in centimeters. In the early stages of cervical effacement, a portion of the cervix

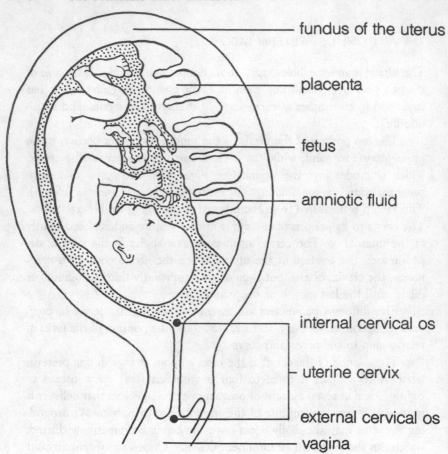

Figure 1. Anatomy of the pregnant uterus.

may not be felt by the examiner, i.e., additional cervix not accessible to the examiner's fingers may be present above the top of the vagina. Therefore, although an examiner's fingers may determine that the cervix is two cm long, or about 40 percent effaced, there may be some additional cervix above the vagina, making the total cervical length three cm. Sometimes an ultrasound measurement of the cervix may provide this additional information. However, as the cervix becomes progressively effaced, this "hidden" cervix disappears rapidly. Because the concept of cervical effacement is a difficult one to grasp, Figure 2 shows some examples.

The *texture* of the pregnant cervix is either firm, moderately soft, or soft. The softer the texture of the cervix, the more likely other changes in the cervix, such as effacement, will occur.

The *angle* of the cervix in the vagina can be a subtle sign of impending cervical effacement and dilation. The more anterior the cervical direction in the vagina (that is, the cervix pointing toward the bladder), the more likely the cervix is to change in other parameters. The more posterior the angle of the cervix (that is, pointing toward the rectum), the more stable the cervix.

The *position of the fetus in the pelvis* in a pregnant woman may have some bearing on the situation of preterm labor. If the presenting part (either the head or the buttocks) of the fetus is "low," it is more likely to contribute to the development of preterm labor, or to aggravate it if it has begun. Figure 3 shows the different positions of the fetus in the pelvis, and also applies to the position of the fetus during normal labor.

If the fetus is at a "0" position at thirty weeks of pregnancy, there is abnormal pressure against the cervix, and this low position may contribute to the development or exacerbation of preterm labor. The Trendelenburg position in bed (hips up, head down) can help to nudge the fetus into a higher position, so that this pressure against the cervix is relieved. (This position is discussed extensively under treatment for premature labor.)

Different practitioners may interpret each cervical parameter differently; two practitioners examining the same cervix may differ as to how much cervical effacement has occurred. However, this difference is usually not great. Often it is important to have only one or two practitioners follow a pregnant patient in preterm labor until the cervix stabilizes, so that the estimation of the cervical parameters is as close as possible.

In general, a cervix that is three cm dilated, 90 percent effaced, soft, anterior, with the fetus at 0 station is in much worse shape in terms of the possibility of a preterm delivery than a cervix that is closed, 50 percent effaced, firm, mid-position, with the fetus at a −2 station. In evaluating the cervix for significant changes, it is also important to take into account the number of weeks of gestation. A cervix with 70 percent effacement at twenty-six weeks is much more worrisome than a cervix 70 percent effaced at thirty-five weeks of gestation. With appropriate treatment, the cervix can re-form to a certain extent (e.g., improvement from 70 percent effaced to 50 percent effaced after a week of treatment).

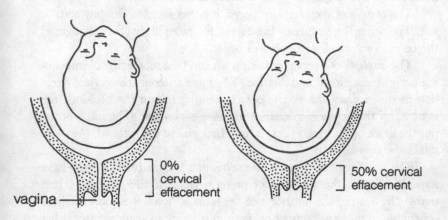

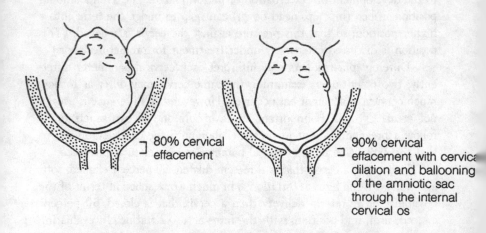

Figure 2. Degrees of cervical effacement.

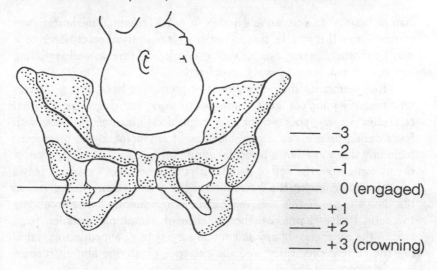

—— -3
—— -2
—— -1
———————————————— 0 (engaged)
—— +1
—— +2
—— +3 (crowning)

Figure 3. Fetal position (station) in the pelvis.

WOMEN AT RISK FOR THE
DEVELOPMENT OF PRETERM LABOR

We are now recognizing that some pregnant women are at higher risk than others for the development of preterm labor. Risk factors for preterm labor existing before the conception of the current pregnancy include a previous preterm labor or preterm delivery, two or more abortions, a history of kidney infections, and a uterus with an abnormal anatomy. Women who have pregnancies before the age of sixteen or after the age of thirty-four are at increased risk for preterm labor, apart from any additional risk factors such as previous abortions.

Another recognized high-risk factor for the development of preterm labor is the exposure of the woman to DES in utero (that is, DES was administered to her mother during pregnancy). DES is an estrogen type of hormone given in the 1950s and 1960s to women who were pregnant and who had indications that they might miscarry. The hormone was given in either pills or injections. If you do not know whether you were exposed to this hormone, and if your mother is living, ask her if she received any medication to help her pregnancy. If she did, try to contact her obstetrician or hospital to determine whether or not a hormonal medication was administered. If it was, be sure to notify your obstetrical practitioner, as it may have other implications for your gynecological care, as well as putting you at high risk for pregnancy complications.

Risk factors for the development of premature labor during the current pregnancy include long commutes to work; smoking more than ten cigarettes per day; poor weight gain; high blood pressure; an illness with fever during pregnancy; vaginal bleeding at any point in the pregnancy, including that caused by a placental abruption (premature pulling away of the placenta from the wall of the uterus); the presence of a placenta previa (the placenta covering the internal os of the cervix, often causing vaginal bleeding and preventing a vaginal birth); extra amniotic fluid surrounding the fetus (polyhydramnios); the presence of a multiple gestation (e.g., twins); the experience of any abdominal surgery (e.g., appendectomy) during the current pregnancy; and the presence of uterine fibroids (benign muscle growths of the uterus).

CAUSES OF PRETERM LABOR

In most cases, a specific cause of preterm labor cannot be found. Different theories have been considered, including a decreased amount of progesterone hormone produced during the pregnancy, the mechanical inability of certain uteri to expand, and the possibility of an excess amount of an adrenalin-like compound (norepinephrine) in the system. However, none of these theories have been proven. In a small number of cases, causes might be detected: an infection inside the uterus around the baby; the presence of an excessive amount of amniotic fluid, putting extra pressure on the uterus; the direct stimulation of the uterus by abdominal surgery. In about 25 percent of pregnant women who develop preterm labor, there is a coexisting "silent" infection of the bladder. Once this infection is treated, the preterm labor can resolve and the pregnant woman may not have a recurrence of the contractions. However, in a significant number of pregnant women with preterm labor and a bladder infection, even if the infection is resolved, preterm labor continues.

It is hoped that in the next few years, the causes of preterm labor will be elucidated. Until then, it is important not to "guilt trip" yourself and think that it was something you "did," such as "working too hard," that caused this condition. It is more important to focus your energy in a positive way toward the treatment of this condition, and not to go over the "what if . . . ?s".

SIGNS OF PREMATURE LABOR

The importance of recognizing the early signs of premature labor cannot be overemphasized. If preterm labor is detected before there is much cervical change, then it is often easily controlled with minimal intervention, e.g., by bedrest alone. However, if early signs are ignored, or cannot be detected, and the pregnant woman in preterm labor arrives with the cervix already significantly dilated, a prolonged hospitalization and multiple medications are often required. In one study, only 20 percent of women in preterm labor were able to receive treatment; 80 percent of the women arriving at the hospital had cervical dilation to such a degree that treatment was not an option. These latter women went on to have premature deliveries.

Recognizing the signs of preterm labor can be difficult, especially for the first-time pregnant woman, as she has never felt uterine contractions before. In contrast to uterine contractions at term, preterm labor contractions are usually painless, and last only twenty to forty seconds. Most women describe preterm contractions as "tightenings," "menstrual type cramping," "gas pains," or the "baby curling up in a ball and staying hard for twenty to sixty seconds." One way to get an idea of what a contraction feels like is to flex your upper arm muscle and to palpate it with the fingers of your opposite hand. The tightening you feel in your flexed arm is similar to that of a uterine contraction.[1] Sometimes it is hard to distinguish between fetal movement and a uterine contraction. Usually the fetal movement lasts only ten to fifteen seconds, versus the twenty to forty seconds for the preterm contractions. You can learn to monitor your own uterus by placing your hand on your uterus. If you feel regular tightenings at a rate of more than two or three per hour, you need to be evaluated for the presence of preterm labor. If you suspect that you may be having an excessive number of uterine contractions, call your obstetrical practitioner. An extra phone call or visit is a small investment compared to waiting until it might be too late to bring the preterm labor under control.

Other symptoms of preterm labor can be vaginal spotting, lower back pain, the loss of the "mucous plug" before the last month, an increase in vaginal discharge, or a feeling of rhythmical pelvic pressure created by a fetus that is being "carried low." Again, because these early signs can be subtle, it is important to check them out as soon as you suspect they may

---

[1] Educational technique developed by premature labor nurses at the University of California Medical Center at San Francisco.

be occurring. Don't wait until you have painful contractions every three minutes; if you wait until then, it may be too late to prevent a premature birth. Don't be afraid that you will be "bothering" your obstetrical practitioner if nothing is found on your exam. Your practitioner will be grateful for an opportunity to diagnose preterm labor on the early side, if it is present.

THE DIAGNOSIS OF PRETERM LABOR

The diagnosis of preterm labor can be very obvious, e.g., a pregnant woman at seven months of pregnancy who has uterine contractions every three minutes, and whose cervix is two cm dilated and 90 percent effaced. On the other hand, the diagnosis of preterm labor can be very subtle, requiring serial evaluations for detection, e.g., a pregnant woman also at seven months of pregnancy who describes occasional uterine tightenings and has 30 percent cervical effacement, and whose contractions increase over the next two days to every twenty minutes with the cervical effacement reaching 50 percent. Both the external uterine monitor and the vaginal exam to evaluate the cervix are used as the cornerstones for the diagnosis of preterm labor.

Once the diagnosis of preterm labor has been made, different tests are often recommended to obtain additional information for decisions as to management. A urine and cervical/vaginal culture are usually ordered to rule out a bladder or vaginal infection. Sometimes blood tests are done, to check for infection and anemia (CBC), and, by measuring blood clotting functions (DIC screen), to check for any evidence of a pulling away of the placenta from the wall of the uterus. Often a baseline ultrasound examination is recommended, to detect any possible cause or associated factor with the preterm labor, e.g., presence of twins or presence of extra amniotic fluid. (See Appendix B for a detailed discussion of monitoring, cultures and ultrasound during pregnancy.)

Once the diagnosis of preterm labor has been established and additional information has been obtained, treatment is initiated. It is important that the treatment be timely, as sometimes a matter of hours may make a difference in the treatment's effectiveness.

TREATMENT OF PREMATURE LABOR

The treatment of premature labor has many components, ranging from simple bedrest to complicated intravenous medications. The type of treatment depends upon many factors, but the overriding considerations are how far the premature labor has progressed, and at how many weeks of gestation the diagnosis is made. With each aspect of treatment, there may be some risks to the mother and/or the fetus, and some possible side effects to both.

Bedrest

In approximately 50 percent of the cases of premature labor that are diagnosed early, the uterine contractions can be controlled with bedrest. Going from the upright position (with gravity "tugging" at the baby) to a prone position (where gravity has no effect of the baby being "pulled downward through the cervix") can in itself relieve the pressure of the baby from the cervix and consequently stop the contractions. However, with the resumption of the upright position the contractions can recur, and so treatment with bedrest must be prolonged.

Bedrest treatment can range from complete (bathroom trips only, with an occasional shower; meals eaten lying down on the side), to partial (in bed two to three hours per day). It is important that you and your partner are clear about the extent of bedrest recommended. This amount can change with each obstetrical visit, as once the premature labor has stabilized small liberties can be granted if the cervix is improved; and vice versa, some activities may be deleted if the cervix or the situation has worsened. Small liberties might include meals at the table for fifteen minutes three times a day, a ten minute walk outside, swimming twice weekly. Greater liberties might include attendance at prepared childbirth class, a dinner out, or a short movie. If you are doing well, establish priorities for your desired activities, and let your practitioner know what they are.

The position of the bed is important in the treatment of preterm labor. If possible, try to elevate the foot of the bed to relieve the pressure of the baby on the cervix. This hip up, head down position is called "Trendelenburg" (see Figure 4). Having pillows under the knees is not helpful, as you have to elevate the hips in order to get the baby to "scoot back" from down in the pelvis toward your chest. It is OK to use one or two pillows for your head, and to turn from side to side. If the bed is a box springs and mattress, you can place a wedge of blankets and sheets between the mattress and the box springs to create the Trendelenburg position. As an alternative, cinder blocks or heavy books may be used to elevate the foot of the bed (or sofa for day use) in the Trendelenburg position.

There are a number of ways to enhance your comfort while lying in this awkward position. An eggcrate mattress is helpful in distributing body

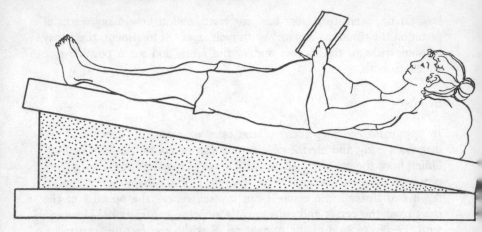

Figure 4. Trendelenburg position of the bed.

pressure and preventing muscle aches from the bedrest. (see Chapter Five, for how to obtain an eggcrate mattress.) The best position for a pregnant woman is not flat on her back, but on either her right or left side (turning frequently to prevent pressure spots on the body, and possibly to prevent one-sided stretch marks!). In the third trimester a small wedge can be used for support underneath the uterus when you are on your side (see Chapter Five for a source for these wedges). Hospital beds are also available for rent, if the above alternatives are not workable. Often medical insurance can help cover the cost of the rental.

Although the most difficult part of bedrest as treatment for preterm labor is usually the psychological coping (see Chapter Two), there may also be physical effects. Bowel function can slow down, making it important to maximize food intake that will encourage smooth bowel function (e.g., bran, whole grains, prunes, salads, lots of liquids). If, despite this extra focus on foods to help constipation, you are having to strain with your bowel movements, you may need to get a stool softener from your practitioner, as straining may cause an increase in pressure on the cervix and therefore an increase in contractions.

Another physical effect from the prolonged bedrest is overall body weakness. The body on bedrest may actually lose muscle mass from all of the inactivity (which may account for poor weight gain by pregnant women on bedrest, although the fetal growth is good). Often women on bedrest experience overwhelming fatigue even doing simple tasks, such as drying their hair. This fatigue is an expected side effect of bedrest. It is important to design a daily exercise program for yourself to try to keep as much strength in your muscles as possible, without jeopardizing the treatment of the preterm labor. Chapter Nine contains exercise guidelines for you.

Another risk of prolonged bedrest is the formation of blood clots in the legs. If you have any varicose veins in your legs, or a history of phlebitis (inflammation of the veins), be sure to ask your practitioner about the use of support hose while on bedrest.

Medication

If bedrest alone is not effective in controlling premature labor, or if the preterm labor has progressed to the point where bedrest alone is not enough, medication is often needed. Certain medications, called "tocolytic" agents, are very effective in stopping the preterm labor contractions by acting directly on the uterus.

In the past, alcohol was used to stop premature labor; however, the levels of alcohol needed to stop the uterine contractions were very high. Mothers who underwent this treatment were quite miserable from continued hangover and vomiting, and of course the high levels of alcohol transmitted to the fetus potentially contributed to the development of fetal alcohol syndrome, with all of its long-term problems for the baby.

At this point in medical history we have four commonly used medications to stop premature labor contractions. These medications may be given orally, by injection, or intravenously.

The only one of the four medications that has been approved by the Federal Drug Administration (FDA) for the specific treatment of premature labor is Ritodrine (Yutopar). Ritodrine has been used for about five years in the United States, and for even longer in Europe. This medication works directly on receptors (proteins) in the uterus that counteract contractions. Unfortunately, there are other organs in the body, such as the heart, with similar receptors, and they are also affected when the medication is taken. Some of the most common side effects of Ritodrine taken orally include an increased heart rate for both the pregnant woman and the fetus, the sensation of pounding of the blood vessels in the head, occasional heart palpitations, headache, nasal congestion, jitteriness, and nausea. These side effects are usually not inherently dangerous in themselves, but can produce some discomfort in the pregnant woman taking the medication. Often these side effects fade in one or two weeks once the body has adjusted to the medication. One of the guidelines most frequently followed to keep the side effects of the medication under control is to guard against the pregnant woman's pulse rate going above 120 beats per minute. If you are having significant side effects from the medication, and especially if your pulse rate is greater than 120, talk with your practitioner. See Glossary (Pulse) for how to measure your pulse.

Ritodrine is usually taken every two hours orally, which means that during the night sleep must be interrupted every two hours. Once the premature labor is under control, the interval between medication doses can be lengthened. Ritodrine is quite expensive, so it is usually worthwhile to call different pharmacies and find the lowest price. Once you have located the pharmacy that you will use, let them know that you need a certain quantity of the medication, as often only a few pills are kept in stock. Also, check with your insurance company to see if the cost of your medication can be covered.

The three other medications commonly used to treat premature labor have not been specifically approved by the FDA for the *treatment of preterm labor*, although they may have been approved for *use in pregnant women* for other conditions, such as asthma or high blood pressure. They have been shown in clinical trials to be effective in stopping premature labor. These medications have been used, for treatment of premature labor, for about ten years both in the United States and Europe, despite the lack of formal FDA approval of these medications for specifically treating preterm labor.

Terbutaline (Brethine) is a medication frequently prescribed to treat premature labor. This medication is also often used for the treatment of asthma, and is much less expensive than Ritodrine. Terbutaline acts on the same receptors as does Ritodrine, with similar side effects. The third medication used to treat premature labor is Vasodilan (Isoxsuprine). This medication has traditionally been used to treat leg cramps caused by narrowed blood vessels. Like the other two medications, it works on the same protein receptors and has similar side effects.

Sometimes a preterm labor patient will respond better to one agent than the other in terms of effectiveness, or will tolerate the side effects more easily. Sometimes more than one medication is used during the treatment of preterm labor. For instance, Ritodrine may have been effective initially for the first two weeks of preterm labor treatment, but the contractions may have recurred. Another medication, e.g., Terbutaline, may now be more effective than the Ritodrine in suppressing the contractions.

If the oral medication is ineffective in stopping the uterine contractions, the usual next step is to administer the medication intravenously (see Appendix B for an explanation of an IV). When the medication is placed through an IV, the dose of the medication to the uterus and its receptors is higher and more continuous, as compared to taking the medication orally. Although the IV medication is extremely effective in treating preterm labor, there are some significant risks.

About 5 percent of pregnant women receiving the IV medication have some serious side effects. These effects can include pulmonary edema (retention of extra fluid in the lungs), an irregular heart beat, and chest pain. Women who are especially at risk for the development of these complications have often had a medical history of heart problems. Be sure to tell your doctor if you have ever had chest pain, rheumatic fever, an irregular heart beat, or a heart murmur. If complications on IV medication are recognized early, they can usually be reversed without long-term consequence to the pregnant woman. Certain precautions are usually taken to minimize these risks. Oral and IV fluid intake are limited (i.e., the amount of juice, milk, and water you drink is measured), and urine output is measured to guard against extra fluid being retained by the body. Routine laboratory tests such as an EKG (an electrical test of the heart, which is a safe procedure during pregnancy) and blood tests are often done to keep track of the body's reaction to the IV medication. The side effects mentioned with the oral medication may be greater in intensity with the IV medication; however, the body often adjusts to these side effects after a few days.

A fourth medication (other than IV Ritodrine, Terbutaline, and Vasodilan) that can be given intravenously is magnesium sulfate. This medication has often been used in the past in pregnant women who have high blood pressure during labor, in order to decrease the chance for the development of seizures. However, this medication also decreases the frequency of uterine contractions. Magnesium sulfate has the same potential risks of the other medications given intravenously, and should be monitored carefully. Regular blood tests to check the concentration of magnesium in the blood are performed.

Once the preterm labor is under control with the IV medications, the dose of the medication is tapered down to a level at which the oral medication can be introduced. During this time of transfer from the IV to the oral medication, it is especially important to be in a quiet environment, and to minimize phone calls and visitors.

What are the possible effects of the medications on the fetus? So far, the effects have been described only with the IV medication. If the baby is born within twenty-four hours of the IV medications, there may be a decreased amount of calcium and glucose in the bloodstream of the baby. This situation can be readily corrected, with those supplements given directly to the baby. The newborn's bowel functions might be slightly slow to begin. However, these are usually minor problems, and most babies exposed to the IV medication have no serious side effects from the medication.

Long-term follow-up studies have been limited. So far, however, after ten years of study, there are no significant differences between those children exposed to the medication and those not exposed. Certainly, if a comparison were made between those children who were exposed to the medication and delivered at term, and those children not exposed to the medication but who were delivered prematurely, the first group would do better in almost every way. As with any medication, the lower the dosage for the mother, the lower the exposure for the fetus. Therefore, it is important to maximize the benefits of bedrest to minimize need for medication. No long-term effects have yet been detected in children exposed to these medications "in utero."

Other Medications Used in the Treatment of Preterm Labor

Occasionally a steroid medication (e.g., betamethasone, dexamethasone) is recommended to the pregnant woman in preterm labor to help accelerate the lung development of the fetus. Its use is controversial, both in terms of its effectiveness in preventing respiratory distress syndrome (immature lungs at birth) and of possible long-term side effects to the fetus (animal studies indicate a possible decrease in organ size, including the brain). The drug should be administered only if there is a strong likelihood of delivery in the next few days. The optimal time of gestation to administer the medication is between twenty-eight and thirty-two weeks. If this medication is recommended to you, be sure to discuss its use in depth with your obstetrician and pediatrician.

Another medication that is sometimes used initially to "calm" the uterus of contractions while the other parts of the premature labor treatment can "take hold" is a narcotic such as morphine. The length of duration of an injection of morphine is six to eight hours. The fetus "naps" along with the pregnant woman, who usually dozes after receiving the medication. If morphine is used only occasionally, there should be no long-term effects on the mother or the fetus.

Sometimes a pregnant woman in preterm labor will have difficulty sleeping at night. Exhaustion can contribute to the exacerbation of preterm uterine contractions. Occasionally Seconal, or Nembutal, are prescribed by your obstetrician for a good night's sleep. As long as delivery is not imminent, there should be no effect on the fetus if this medication is used only occasionally. Some pregnant women find an amino acid, L-tryptophan, to be helpful in obtaining a good night's sleep. This tablet can be found at health food stores.

If a bladder or vaginal infection is present, antibiotics are sometimes prescribed. The treatment of these concomitant infections is very important. Only antibiotics that have been approved for use in pregnancy are routinely used. These antibiotics may include Ampicillin, Keflex, Erythromycin, or Anspor.

Although all pregnant women and medical practitioners prefer that no medication at all be given during a pregnancy, one has to assess the risks of a certain situation and weigh the benefits of the medications. It is far preferable for a pregnant woman in preterm labor to receive one or two medications than to have to administer up to twenty-two different medications to the premature baby who would be born if the premature labor were not stopped. The best nursery, in almost all circumstances, is the mother's womb.

Hospitalization and the
Treatment of Preterm Labor

Although occasionally preterm labor can be diagnosed and treated in an outpatient setting, the initial evaluation and treatment often occurs in a hospital. Hospitals can be overwhelming, especially to a couple who have little experience with them and were looking forward to being in the hospital setting only at the time of a normal, full-term birth. Chapter Six explores the hospital experience and has many helpful hints on how to deal with it.

If the preterm labor is easily controlled initially in the hospital, then the pregnant woman can often go home after a few days. However, if there is difficulty in treating the preterm labor, then often a transfer to a hospital with an Intensive Care Nursery is considered, if the original hospital does not have one.

Hospital nurseries are classified according to the level of care that is offered to newborns. Most hospitals have Level I nurseries, which means that they have facilities to care for full-term newborns, including those with mild complications, such as jaundice. Usually Level I nurseries can comfortably care for the mildly premature baby (over thirty-three weeks gestation at birth). If a baby of less than thirty-three weeks is delivered at a hospital with a Level I nursery, and the premature infant has problems, such as respiratory difficulties, a transfer is then arranged to a Level II or a Level III nursery (the Level I nursery has the equipment and personnel to stabilize the baby initially). A Level II nursery is capable of caring for a wide range of premature infants, and is staffed with a full-time neonatologist (a pediatrician with special training in the care of newborns with problems). A Level III nursery is usually found only in large cities, and is often affiliated with a university. This nursery is staffed by many specialists, such as pediatric heart surgeons. Level III nurseries care for the premature baby or full-term newborn with severe medical or surgical problems.

If a premature birth is imminent, it is important that the pregnant woman deliver in the appropriate facility. If she is stable enough this may require an ambulance transfer (if that facility is not at the original hospital). The long-term outcome for premature babies is influenced by the availability of expert care from the first moment of birth. Even if a transfer to another facility might mean an unknown hospital and obstetrician, it is important to remember that the care of the premature newborn must be regarded as a very critical issue.

LABOR AND DELIVERY OF PREGNANT WOMEN WHO HAVE BEEN SUCCESSFULLY TREATED FOR PRETERM LABOR

Once you have reached thirty-seven or thirty-eight weeks of gestation, the medication and bedrest are discontinued, unless another pregnancy complication has occurred, such as high blood pressure requiring continued bedrest. A few pregnant women previously on bedrest will deliver in the first few days after resuming normal activity; however, the majority will continue on to thirty-eight to forty weeks of pregnancy, as the uterus has become tolerant of contractions that two months ago may have meant that delivery was imminent. Occasionally a woman who has had preterm labor delivers past her due date. This prolongation of pregnancy usually means that the event initiating her preterm labor has resolved, and her uterus is following the pattern of the 50 percent of women who do not experience preterm labor who deliver after their due date.

There have been no extensive studies of the labor patterns of women who have been successfully treated for preterm labor during the pregnancy. However, we have made several anecdotal observations. In women who have undergone premature cervical effacement, the latent or prodromal phase of labor seems to be shortened by several hours (the latent phase is made up of the early hours of labor when the effacement and early dilation of the cervix are occurring). Some women who have undergone multiple premature labor contractions are afraid that they will not recognize "real" labor when it happens, as they often have regular uterine contractions. *Don't worry!* You *will* be able to recognize labor. The contractions are very regular, e.g., every three to five minutes, they last forty to sixty seconds from beginning to end, and you will have to use your breathing techniques with these contractions—you won't be able to talk through them.

Most obstetricians consider patients who have been treated for premature labor and who are now at term to be at high risk during labor. After all, because the cause of the premature labor is often unknown, a "hidden" cause might surface during labor. For instance, a tiny placental abruption (see Glossary) that was impossible to detect by ultrasound may have initiated the preterm labor. This same tiny abruption might extend during the labor at term and cause fetal distress. Therefore, most obstetricians recommend external monitoring during the active labor of a patient who has previously been treated for premature labor during her pregnancy, to detect fetal distress.

However, being monitored does not need to interfere with your personal birth plans. Some hospitals allow monitoring in Alternative Birthing Rooms, if your obstetrician is comfortable with your delivery there. Even if your physician recommends delivery in the most traditional of settings, individual birth plans can still be followed, e.g., immediate holding of the baby and breastfeeding. Remember, it is not the physical surroundings but the attitudes of the people at the birth that create the warm, caring atmosphere into which your baby will be born. You have worked *so* hard to give your baby a healthy start! Don't let the presence or absence of details in your birth plan interfere with the principal goal of guiding your baby through a safe labor!

As a group, women who have been treated for preterm labor in their pregnancies often have a higher rate of Cesarean births than women who have problem-free pregnancies. While not all of the reasons are clear, it is known that women with placenta previa and placental abruptions have a significant risk of premature labor. Therefore, these reasons probably contribute to the increased rate of Cesarean sections in this group. *All* women in labor should be prepared for the possibility of a Cesarean section, e.g., for unexpected fetal distress. However, remember that your chances of a vaginal delivery *are* probably over 50 percent! Try to be prepared no matter what happens.

Post-partum courses of women treated for preterm labor seem to be similar to those of women with uncomplicated pregnancies. However, the weeks of bedrest may have taken a toll on body strength, and post-partum fatigue may be increased. It often seems that psychologically, families who experience preterm labor feel "liberated" once the birth has occurred, while their counterparts are just realizing how "tied down" they are now with the arrival of a new family member after a problem-free pregnancy!!!

FUTURE PREGNANCIES ONCE PRETERM LABOR HAS OCCURRED

Once you have experienced preterm labor in one pregnancy, you are at risk for this complication during your next pregnancy, and you need to be observed carefully in order to detect a recurrence of preterm labor. The estimated risk for the recurrence of preterm labor with a subsequent pregnancy is between 25 percent to 50 percent. If the preterm labor was initiated by a definite event, such as an appendectomy, then the chances of recurrence are lower. If the reason for the preterm labor was an abnormal shape of the uterus, then the chances are higher. However, because in the majority of the cases of preterm labor a cause cannot be found, the risk of a recurrence of preterm labor in a future pregnancy is usually considered to be between 25 percent to 50 percent.

ELYSA'S STORY

While dressing for work when I had just reached my thirty-fourth week of pregnancy, I first began to feel cramping at the lower part of my stomach. I passed it off as nothing serious, as I still had six weeks until my due date. I proceeded to go to work and nonchalantly called my doctor, and before I knew it, I was in my doctor's office on a fetal monitor. After several contractions showed up on the reading, the doctor ordered complete bedrest for the next four weeks. Everything seemed to have happened so quickly— explanations of why and what was happening inside me, instructions for my care, prescriptions, appointments; not to mention that my life took a major and unexpected change much sooner than I had psyched myself for. Once I got myself settled, my husband and I slowly worked ourselves into a routine. I felt badly for him, working all day and then coming home to care for me. But we took it on, with no questions asked—it was a team effort. My family lived three thousand miles away. They called often, and were scared and confused. Each member had such longing in their voices. My mother called once or twice a day. Sometimes her phone calls were such a welcome relief, while others were difficult. The difficult ones were because she so much wanted to be with me and was unable to do so. Dealing with my situation was almost harder on her than it was on me.

At night I had severe anxiety attacks that would wake me at two or three o'clock in the morning. I felt as though I had baby up to my neck and couldn't breathe. When would this all be over? The medication, the bedrest, the helplessness, the loneliness. My husband would wake up with me and calm me down and comfort me back into a somewhat sound sleep. I never had a good night's sleep during that time. There was so much turmoil in my mind with my job and my family, and of course the outcome of the health of this baby.

I also began to stop thinking of this baby as a baby—boy or girl—but as a condition. I know now that if this were to happen to me again with my next pregnancy, I would accept it more willingly, knowing now and having experienced the marvel of birth and the feeling of loving a child.

The premature labor was finally controlled by both the bedrest and medication. By thirty-eight weeks of pregnancy, I was allowed my normal activity. Having just experienced the anxiety of premature labor, I was about to face the further frustration of delivering eleven days beyond my due date.

My mind was reeling with so many more thoughts and emotions than I've expressed here, but one thing always stands out as I recall that time in my life. It didn't occur to me until after the birth of my daughter how incredibly important it was for the baby to go full term. What had appeared to be only sleepless nights, endless days, physical discomfort, and loneliness, in retrospect is a small price of ourselves to pay for the really wonderful experience of being parents.

Elysa Waldholz-Goldblatt,
mother of Jamie (one year).

WEAKENED OR "INCOMPETENT" CERVIX

At sixteen weeks of pregnancy, I began to notice a definite pressure in my lower uterus, similar to the feeling I would get before my period started. I went in for a checkup, and learned that my cervix had begun silently to efface. Because bedrest didn't help, I had a suture placed in my cervix. I keep guilt-tripping myself that my cervix was weak because of the three abortions I had had earlier. But my practitioner says that this condition can also hap-

*pen to women who have never been pregnant. Thank
goodness there is a treatment!*

> A woman who delivered
> after her cerclage was
> removed at thirty-eight weeks.

The term "incompetent cervix" is an unfortunate one, as it disparages a part of the body which, through no fault of its own, is weak relative to the weight of the fetus, placenta, and amniotic fluid. The proper term should be a "weakened" cervix, not incompetent cervix. Therefore, while traditional medical terminology has described this condition as an incompetent cervix, "weakened cervix" will be used throughout this chapter.

By definition a weakened cervix is one that progressively effaces and/ or dilates without the presence of uterine contractions. The classical time of the diagnosis is between sixteen to twenty-two weeks of pregnancy. However, the condition can occur at any time during the pregnancy. The detection is based on the same five parameters used in the evaluation of premature labor: effacement, dilation, consistency of the cervix; the axis of the cervix in the vagina; and the depth of the presenting part of the fetus in the pelvis. However, unlike premature labor, there are no regular uterine contractions to accompany these cervical changes.

Certain women are at higher risk than others for developing a weakened cervix. Risk factors include a history of multiple D & Cs (dilation and curretage) in the past (whether for abortion or other reasons), exposure to DES in utero (discussed earlier in this chapter), and previous surgery on the cervix (e.g., cervical conization for an abnormal Pap smear). A few years ago, before the risk factors were recognized and women at risk were examined more frequently, a common history for these women was a sudden second-trimester pregnancy loss (e.g., arriving at labor and delivery with only a feeling of pelvic pressure, to discover that the cervix was already ten cm dilated and that nothing could be done to stop the impending miscarriage). However, now that we can identify women who are at risk for developing this condition, this type of sudden pregnancy loss occurs less frequently, as the condition is often diagnosed early enough so that preventive measures can be taken.

Occasionally, women with no risk factors at all can develop a weakened cervix. Therefore all pregnant women should be aware of any signs of a weakened cervix, and should report them to their clinician immediately. They can include vaginal spotting (light bleeding), a feeling of pelvic pressure, menstrual-type cramping, increased vaginal discharge, or the development of a mucousy discharge. Because these signs can be very subtle, it is important that each be evaluated by the obstetrical practitioner and not be ignored as something minor. It is far better to make extra obstetrical visits than to shrug off some of these early findings and wait until it is too late to save the pregnancy.

The diagnosis of a weakened cervix depends, for the most part, on progressive cervical effacement and dilation over a period of time that is not accompanied by uterine contractions. Besides serial cervical examinations to establish the diagnosis, external uterine monitoring is often used to rule out any component of premature labor contributing to the cervical changes. Sometimes ultrasound helps to establish the diagnosis of weakened cervix. With an ultrasound, the cervix can be measured in centimeters and an assessment of the amniotic sac made, to determine whether or not it is "ballooning" down through the internal cervical canal.

Treatment of the weakened cervix can range from bedrest, to the insertion of a pessary (a diaphragm-like ring placed in the vagina to elevate the uterus), to the placement of a suture in the cervix (cervical cerclage).

Bedrest can be effective in relieving the pressure on the cervix of the fetus, the placenta, and the amniotic fluid. In some cases the relief of the pressure allows the cervix to re-form to a certain extent (e.g., from 70 percent effaced and soft, to 40 percent effaced and moderately firm). The Trendelenburg position may be an important factor in this treatment (see Figure 4 for a description of bedrest in Trendelenburg position). Occasionally a pessary is inserted into the vagina to take the pressure of the uterus off the cervix (see Figure 5). Sometimes with the pessary only partial bedrest is necessary.

If a cervical cerclage (suture of the cervix) is necessary, the cerclage is placed under anesthesia at the hospital. One way to understand a cerclage and what it does is to imagine a purse with a drawstring on the top. When the two ends of the drawstring are pulled tightly, the purse is closed and its contents cannot spill. A cerclage is a "purse-string" suture placed in the cervix; a knot is tied after it is in place to assure that the contents of the uterus are held tightly within.

Most cerclages are of the "McDonald" type, and are removed two to three weeks before the due date. A vaginal delivery is then anticipated, barring unforeseen problems. However, sometimes a more complicated suture is necessary, for instance when the cervix is anatomically unsuited for a McDonald cerclage; this more complicated suture is called the Shirodkar. The Shirodkar suture is usually permanent, and thus a Cesarean section is required for delivery.

The cerclage is placed under anesthesia, as it is essential that the pregnant woman not move during its placement. Most anesthesiologists

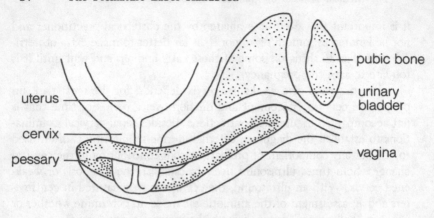

uterus

cervix

pessary

pubic bone

urinary
bladder

vagina

Figure 5. Pessary.

use either spinal anesthesia or epidural anesthesia, as only a minimal amount of medication, if any, is transmitted to the growing fetus with this type of anesthesia. However, in certain cases a general anesthetic is used. (See Appendix B for a more detailed description of anesthesia.)

The risk of complications from the placement of a cerclage is less than 5 percent. Possible risks include premature leaking of amniotic fluid (usually resolved with bedrest), replacement of the suture if it weakens after several months (usually done easily), vaginal bleeding (which usually resolves spontaneously), and possible infection developing around the baby. (This complication of infection is quite rare; however, if it does occur, immediate delivery is indicated.)

Occasionally, two sutures instead of one are placed at the time of the surgery if the cervix is technically difficult to close. Complications leading to loss of the pregnancy because of the cerclage procedure are in the 1 to 2 percent range. After the cerclage is in place, the pregnant woman is usually observed closely for several hours. It is important to be certain that no premature contractions are "stirred up" by the stimulation of the cervix during the placement of the stitch.

After discharge from the hospital, the patient with the cerclage is checked frequently, and varying amounts of bedrest may be prescribed. Because patients with a cerclage in place are at high risk for the development of premature labor, these women should be especially aware of any

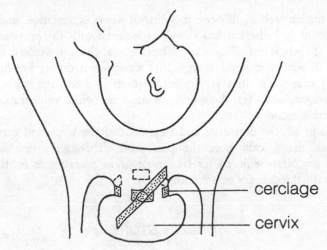

Figure 6. McDonald Cerclage.

of the early symptoms of premature labor, such as painless uterine tightening, vaginal spotting, etc.

Sometimes cervical effacement and dilation can be due to a combination of premature labor and a weakened cervix, and both a cerclage and medication for the premature labor are required for the pregnancy to continue.

If a weakened cervix is diagnosed early (e.g., before the cervix is greater than two to three cm dilated and 90 percent effaced), pregnant women who are treated usually do quite well and continue their pregnancies to term. Once the pregnancy is at term and the cerclage is removed, it is advisable for the pregnant woman to walk around the area for a couple of hours and to be checked internally again, as labor may begin within a few hours. However, most pregnancies continue for a week or two longer after the cerclage is removed. Very occasionally there may be some scarring from the suture that might interfere with progressive cervical dilation in labor, and a Cesarean section may be required for the delivery.

Once a woman has been diagnosed with a weakened cervix during the pregnancy, she is at risk for this condition to recur during her next pregnancy. However, during the next pregnancy, the cerclage is usually placed preventively at thirteen to fourteen weeks of gestation, and often the amount of bedrest is less than was required with the previous pregnancy (as there is less dilation and effacement at thirteen weeks compared to the amount of cervical change that was present during her first cerclage). Occasionally, in a very difficult situation, a cerclage is placed *between* pregnancies. (Yes, the sperm are small enough to swim through the purse-string suture!)

All in all, the detection and treatment of the weakened cervix has improved dramatically over the past years. Although a cerclage and bedrest are often required for treatment, most pregnancies continue to term, with the delivery of a healthy baby.

CINDY'S STORY

I had planned one of those drug and alcohol-free pregnancies, expecting to look like the pregnant women in the movies—great clothes, exercising until the end, etc. Well, my problems began at eleven weeks, possibly stemming from my exposure to DES in utero, which my mother took when she was pregnant with me, in order to avoid a miscarriage. The problems continued for twenty-three weeks, with cervical effacement due to an incompetent cervix, a subsequent cerclage, and four trips to the hospital to control premature labor, in addition to round-the-clock doses of Ritodrine or Terbutaline. Despite all this, we produced a healthy baby!

We feel that the most important aspect of our success was having complete confidence in my physicians and following their instructions to the letter. We developed a positive outlook on everything, holding onto any positive comments from my obstetricians. We set goals of twenty, twenty-eight, and thirty-two weeks, and were looking toward thirty-six weeks when our son was born. This allowed us periodic feelings of accomplishment, as forty weeks just seemed decades away. We also considered my trips to the hospital as "vacations," knowing that I would be well taken care of and my being away would give my husband Bill a night "off."

We spent time together every night doing what we called "P.E.T." or Positive Energy Transfer. We would put our hands on my abdomen and concentrate on all the anatomical systems of the baby's body, visualizing each as perfect. This technique also helped slow down the contractions at times and calmed me when my pulse was accelerated because of the drugs. We reassured ourselves that the side effects of the medication were temporary, and that they were necessary.

I kept myself busy for five months in bed by doing crossword puzzles, reading, and daydreaming. Because I couldn't exercise, I visualized running by the ocean, feeling the wind on my face and the exhaustion of my muscles. This I did every day. I've never run so well or so fast! Mail was greatly appreciated, although phone calls were kept to a minimum—every ring of the phone meant a contraction! I also kept a journal, and moved from the bedroom to the living room for a change of scenery.

I was able to attend only three Lamaze classes—lying down, of course —but found that I delivered just fine without the rest of them. My plans for an ABC (Alternative Birth Center) delivery were thwarted by the early arrival of our baby. I took consolation in the fact that at least my labor was only five hours long, and that his birth was a relaxed and natural event.

Christopher was born without any major complications at thirty-four weeks of gestation. (An amniocentesis performed the day before the birth had determined that his lungs were fully mature.) Some routine procedures used on him in the nursery were confusing to my husband, as we hadn't had time to consult our pediatrician about techniques used on premature infants. We *strongly* recommend an *early* consultation with a pediatrician and thorough questioning of medical procedures. We were unnecessarily concerned about an intravenous line in his umbilicus and an oxygen hood. We feel that this anxiety could have been prevented with a bit more information.

Because he was premature, Chris was unable to suck. I began using an electric breast pump every three hours at home, and in the nurse's locker room at the hospital during my visits there. Chris stayed at the hospital for three weeks until he reached four-and-a-half pounds. He tolerated my breast milk much better than the formula he was given the first day, which made me feel that I was contributing to his health, even though he wasn't at home with us. He didn't learn to nurse until he was six weeks old —frustrating at times, but *absolutely* worth the indignity of hooking up to a machine. I am glad I persevered!

Other than my lack of muscle tone and a significant weight gain, I suffered no physiological repercussions from my pregnancy. Christopher is two years old, and we are ready to go through it again, as it is *definitely* worth it. We have forgotten the frustration and look forward to having another child in the near future—as soon as we three conquer the potty!!!

Cindy P. Gates, mother of Christopher (two years).

2

THE STRESSES
OF PREMATURE LABOR

*I finally burned out on telling myself I was "lucky" or
trying to view this as an "opportunity" to learn something. To hell with being a good girl-patient-mother. I
almost put my fist through the wall.*

Expectant Mother

*Talk about it? Talk about it?! I don't have time to talk
about it! What I need is someone to come help me wash
the floor!*

Expectant Father

No one needs to tell you that you're both undergoing a great deal of stress.
No special insight is necessary to acknowledge that sudden confinement
and dependency for one of you, double duty at home and work for the
other, and financial and sexual losses for both, is a lot to have descend all
at once. And then, of course, there's your overriding concern about your
baby. Premature labor is a critical event fraught with multiple stresses.
Some are fairly self-evident; others emerge unexpectedly. Some affect everyone in your position to one degree or another; some are unique to your
personal situation and makeup.

What might be helpful to hear from someone else, beginning with this chapter, is (1) how the common stressors[1] have affected other people, (2) what some of the more subtle stressors can be, and (3) some first-hand strategies for coping. We will address these issues as they usually affect the woman in premature labor, her partner, and the couple relationship. We urge you both to read each section and to share with one another what hit home for you. Also, if you choose to do so, note the stressors that currently affect you in the first column of the worksheet at the end of this chapter. You may use the worksheet to devise coping strategies as outlined later.

COMMON SOURCES OF STRESS

WORRY ABOUT THE BABY

> *There I was, lying in the labor room at twenty-four weeks in my pregnancy, giggling so uncontrollably that we could hardly get a monitor reading of my contractions. They gave me morphine, then Nembutal, and I still could not sleep. One week later, with the contractions still not under control, we began to confront what we might do if our baby were born so early. I could not stand to face it at first, and then I had to imagine the worst just to convince myself that I could cope.*
>
> *Expectant Mother*

For many couples the first worry when they hear "premature labor," and the most persistent one up to the time of birth, is whether the baby is healthy. This worry may be acute at the beginning if the diagnosis and orders to bed are relatively sudden and unexpected. If the woman's activity has been restricted more gradually, the worry may emerge more slowly. It is fairly safe to say that for all women in premature labor, and for their partners as well, there will be some measure of anxiety, some measure of denial, and some measure of ambivalence.

Anxiety may show up in a number of ways. You may at times feel outright fear about early delivery and about your baby's chances for survival and health. Your attention may be attracted to media presentations

---

[1] In this chapter we shall use the term "stressor" to denote events or phenomena. The term "stress" shall be used to refer to the internal response to such stressors.

on prematurity. You may be subject to extremes of uncontrollable tears or laughter, even cracking a few "sick" jokes here or there. Many patients report fears that their baby may die. Such fears will be exacerbated if you have had a previous miscarriage. You may find yourself reliving in your mind a past loss. Such imaginings frequently serve to provide a sense of control over the situation; by replaying the past, you may search for clues pertaining to the present. Alternatively, by reliving a past loss, you may be able to mourn more fully and to lay it to rest, enabling you to engage the present circumstance as a new and separate event. If you are one for whom feelings about a previous pregnancy loss reemerge, you may want to consult some of the excellent sources of support listed in the Bibliography.

On the other hand, you may find yourself imagining the worst for the future. By anticipating the future, one psychologically "prepares" and reassures oneself that coping is possible. In any case, your fears are important and certainly to be expected. More will be said below about understanding and expressing them. Your clinician will have advised you if there are reasons other than early labor to feel cautious about your baby's health. If you have any remaining questions, ask your obstetrical practitioner. Perhaps one of the best ways to reassure yourselves is to keep in mind that such fears are, indeed, quite common among those whose pregnancies have been threatened, and even among couples who have not had difficulties with their pregnancy. The overwhelming majority of these pregnancies result in healthy children. Solicit such success stories from your clinician and hold them in mind.

As a woman in premature labor, you may become preoccupied with bodily details. You will question whether what you just experienced was a contraction or a gas pain. You will note the baby's every movement or lack thereof, your weight gain or lack thereof. You may feel utterly at the mercy of this expanding involuntary muscle called your uterus, and of your effaceable cervix, leading you to feel "oh so fragile." At the other end of the spectrum, you may at times feel oppressively powerful, as if your every move—or worse yet, *thought*—may make a difference.

If you are the partner of a woman in premature labor, your preoccupation will be less complete simply because you have so much else to do, but your worry will probably be no less. In the same way that a woman tries to master worry by gaining some kind of control (and hence can become absorbed by her bodily experiences), you too will look for sources of information and control. However, since the baby is not within you, you have fewer ready-made aspects upon which to focus. Therefore, your signs of worry may be more indirect. You may focus on your partner's eating, sleeping, or movement habits as things over which you can at least try to have some influence. You may turn to career, home, or financial issues as an outlet for your concern. Your worry about the baby may be direct and acute only during or immediately following times of "crisis."

Fortunately, you both have the healthy mechanism of denial also at work for you. There are other things to pour yourselves into. Many remark with surprise that they have not felt worried to any great degree. Others feel the worry periodically lift and then return. In either case, you probably need not be concerned that you are "not facing reality." Denial is one way your psyche protects, relieves, and refuels itself. You may even find yourself questioning whether all these precautions are necessary, and skewing the clinician's information toward the positive side. If, however, you find yourself significantly discounting and disregarding your medical practitioner's information and advice regarding your treatment, request a meeting to explore the reasoning behind the recommended treatment. At times a more complete understanding of your clinician's recommendations can make them seem more worthwhile. At other times, changes in your treatment may be negotiated, making it more suitable to your needs. If all else fails, a second opinion may help you to evaluate the situation, and offer reassurance or provide more options for you. Finally, when sorting through your feelings about the pregnancy and the anxiety that has been caused by your premature labor condition, you may find that consultation with a professional psychotherapist may be of invaluable assistance as well.

While anxiety about the baby's safety is common and "speakable," ambivalence toward the baby is also common, and frequently feels "unspeakable." Mixed emotions about the baby may range from mildly resentful hopes that this child will appreciate everything you've done, to outright questioning of whether the sacrifices are worth it, and overt anger at the baby. This is especially true for women confined to bed with other young children at home. They describe being torn between one child and the next in a way that is difficult to reconcile. It seems to be especially true for partners as well. Partners frequently feel somewhat abandoned by their mates when a baby is born. The confinement of premature labor can seem to accelerate this sense of abandonment as your mate, even sooner than expected, is not as available for your previously enjoyed joint activities. Some of the resentment this causes can predictably be expected to focus upon the baby.

Of course, ambivalence is a natural result of feeling torn between any two things one loves—career and your baby, physical activity and your baby, your mate and your baby. Throughout the premature labor experience both of you are bound to feel mixed emotions toward all these realms of your life. What you feel today is probably not fixed. By allowing yourself to experience and acknowledge your various emotions—and perhaps by finding some way to do so with each other—you will move through them more quickly and with greater understanding.

Two feelings that frequently accompany anxiety about the baby (especially for the woman in premature labor) are responsibility and guilt. You search for reasons or causes for this situation, and if medical personnel can't provide them, you may tend to turn to your own behavior, thoughts, or attitudes. We noted in Chapter One some ways in which women in premature labor may "guilt-trip" themselves regarding possible precursors to their condition. *And* we noted the futility and nonproductivity of rehashing these "what if . . . ?s." The same holds true of looking for psychological precursors to premature labor. We do know that in some cases, when premature labor has already been initiated, stress can cause contractions. You will note this yourself, as you monitor your own activity and emotional responses. One cannot, however, conclude that emotional stressors *caused* the original premature labor. It has been suggested that severe and multiple psychological and social stressors are *associated* with complications of pregnancy. However, such studies are so fraught with difficulties of study design as to render any conclusion about *causation* of the problems virtually impossible. That is, in order to conclude that a woman's emotional state contributes significantly to a difficulty in pregnancy requires first ruling out all medical and physical factors, all considerations of her prenatal care, nutrition, and environmental conditions. We know of no studies to date that include all these variables. We also know that many women who have undergone rather severe emotional distress have uncomplicated, full-term pregnancies.

You may find yourself sorting through your attitudes and feelings over the past months to find some cause for your situation. In a word, *don't*—if the purpose of that search is solely to establish responsibility and guilt. Blaming yourself for feeling ambivalent about the pregnancy or for having stressors in your life is unproductive. If, however, such an examination is prompted by your wish to look at the meaning of this event in your life, and if it includes psychological or attitudinal factors, examine away. But do be compassionate with yourself. A search for meaning is different from a search for blame. You will find that this premature labor experience invites a lot of self-examination. That, indeed, can be one of its gifts, if you look inward openly and positively.

As your treatment progresses, you may find yourself at times feeling oppressively responsible for promoting a good outcome. You may feel as if your baby's fate hinges upon your movements, your moods, anything that can cause a contraction. You may feel guilty about not always being "good," about that "illegal" trip to get something you wanted, about your resentment and mixed feelings. Knowing that others also experience these things may ease your sense that you should be doing better. Still, the truth is that housing and nourishing your baby *is* a tremendous responsibility. Acknowledging this in its positive sense may lend meaning to those times when you mistakenly interpret your reduced activity as "doing nothing."

Coping with Worry About the Baby

Worry is the result of not knowing whether a feared outcome will come to pass. It can be worsened by not talking about it, allowing it to fester and spread. It can be worsened by trying to avoid or postpone looking at the reality of possible outcomes. It can also be worsened by dwelling too much on the future to the exclusion of your current reality.

Talking about your individual fears may be difficult either because you are not ready to say them out loud or because you don't want to make someone else worry—or both. The truth is that speaking your fears will not make them happen, and many of your loved ones are probably already harboring the same fears. It is also true that you may need to be somewhat selective about when and to whom you voice those concerns. Not everyone in your usual support circle will be able to be supportive at this time, for their own emotionally based reasons, and there will be times, especially with your partner, when talking is not easy.

Talking to each other about your worries can be one of the most consoling things you can do. It can also pose a challenge if your cycles of denial and anxiety are out of sync. Sometimes you won't want to hear about your partner's worry or, conversely, your partner may seem impatient or callous. Recognizing your respective stages in the coping process can help you to feel less at odds with each other at those times. At other times you may find that when you are not in your own worry mode, you are better able to listen to and support your partner.

Invariably, couples find that clear and frequent information about available medical treatment options and (as far as possible) information about the probabilities of various outcomes is a tremendous help in combatting fearful fantasies. It may be helpful too to remember that you are in bed because obstetrics is indeed getting better at detecting early labor and preventing premature birth. If you have not already heard some, ask your medical practitioner to share with you stories of other couples who have been in premature labor and delivered healthy babies. If possible, arrange to speak with some of them yourself. Also, consider the following facts:

— Often women who are diagnosed early and who are put to bed with premature labor carry their babies to full term.

— The probabilities of health for a baby delivered by a mother who experienced premature labor and reached full term are approximately the same as those for a baby whose mother experienced no premature labor.

— There are no known long-term negative effects upon the baby from the medications (other than ethanol) commonly employed to control premature labor.

At some point, many couples find it a relief to inform themselves about the realities of premature birth. Parents frequently ask the following kinds of questions:

— What are the baby's chances for survival and health?
— What might the complications be?
— What factors are to be weighed in determining these things?
— Where would the baby be treated?
— How would we be allowed contact with the baby?
— What would the baby look like?

Chapter Seven begins to address these questions. A number of good additional sources of information are available as well. The first, of course, is your medical practitioner. Viewing a film on prematurity and talking with pediatricians and parents of a premature baby may also be helpful. As a start, we have included a bibliography of information on prematurity at the end of this book.

Although anticipating the possible future is an inevitable and important process, staying in touch with your baby and yourselves right now is essential. There are many books on the market that describe fetal development and allow you to keep abreast of your baby's milestones week by week (see the Bibliography). Each week that the baby is in utero is a major step toward health. The baby's lungs develop and weight is gained. Indeed, your baby's growth is still the miraculous and joyous process that it was in the early weeks of your pregnancy. Chapter Ten suggests some ways for tuning in to your baby through thought, visualization, and touch. By following these suggestions you may feel a greater kinship with your baby while sustaining your pregnancy.

BONNIE'S STORY

Dan and I planned for this baby and looked forward to natural childbirth, the ABC room, the works! Our dreams were not to materialize. . . . I had an easy and wonderful pregnancy until I began my third trimester; then my blood pressure began to rise and I had protein in my urine. We were living in Northern California and planned to move to Los Angeles before our baby's due date (Dan and I both grew up there, so we were "coming home"). My obstetrician suggested we make the move as soon as my blood pressure began to rise. I had my first appointment with a new medical group two months before I was due. My new doctors put me on total bedrest (on my left side—this position increases blood flow, oxygen, and nutrition to the baby), and began a series of lab tests, hospitalizations, ultrasounds, amniocentesis (three in all), nonstress tests, oxytocin challenge tests, etc. That was to go on for seven weeks, until Rachel was finally born.

I'll spare you the gory details. Mostly I'd like to talk about the way I felt during those seven weeks in bed and at the beginning of Rachel's life. We had an added stress since we had just moved (I supervised the move while lying on my left side on a mattress on the front lawn), Dan was starting a new business association, and I was starting with new doctors (they were a blessing, worried and depressed as I was).

I followed the doctors' orders religiously, as I felt I had no choice about it—but I sure did feel sorry for myself! My primary feeling was constant worry about the life and health of our baby. The doctors sent me for what seemed like endless ultrasounds to determine whether or not she was growing (her growth had been too slow, because of my high blood pressure), and they explained IUGR (Intra Uterine Growth Retardation) to us. I was terrified that our child's brain would be underdeveloped, and I was scared that maybe she wouldn't make it at all. In addition, I was concerned about my own health—how dangerous was it for me to have such high blood pressure, even just for a few months; would the pregnancy cause permanent kidney damage . . . ? Towards the end, I was taking medication for premature labor contractions (Ritodrine)—and I had wanted to have a drug-free, caffeine-free pregnancy! Then I began to worry about the effects of the drug on my baby.

I had a hard time accepting my total dependence on others to do everything for me—my husband, our families, and friends really came through and helped in every way they could. I felt guilty that Dan had to do all the household chores, after all the years of our sharing everything. The experiences we had brought Dan and me even closer—we shared the fear, the worry, and the limitations on me.

On July 12, I went to the hospital for my regular nonstress test and didn't return home! Rachel was born the next day, after the third amniocentesis showed that her lungs were finally mature. The relief of the pregnancy finally being over was replaced by worry about the tiny, fragile child we now had. She had to stay in the hospital isolette for two weeks, until she weighed four lbs. The third day of Rachel's life I finally fell apart emotionally from the incredible strain I had been under—now the reality of my baby, alive and physically healthy, but with the question of the possible growth retardation, hit me. My doctor, who was on call and in the hospital, came immediately when Dan told her of my condition. She listened to me, comforted me, and reassured me that my reaction was normal and understandable.

Now that we had our baby, the normal insecurities of first-time parents became exaggerated by worries about her development. She gained weight rapidly, but our pediatrician said we couldn't know about her brain development until she was between six and eighteen months old. I read all the baby books and compared her to all the other babies. I desperately wanted to see that she was developing at a normal rate. By the time Rachel was nine months old, I knew in my heart that she was developing at a perfectly normal rate and that she had caught up in all ways.

I hope none of us ever has to go through such a traumatic time again. I also hope that my experience provides you with some comfort and hope. We have an incredible daughter now—yes, she was worth it. Yet, I'm still not sure that I would go through it again . . . that's a very hard decision for me to make. . . .

> *Bonnie Ziveta Silverman, mother*
> *of Rachel (three years).*

CHANGES IN YOUR USUAL LIFE ROLES

One of you is trying to do so much less, the other so much more. Like Jack and Ms. Spratt, you try to strike a new and satisfying balance. It probably took you a considerable time to evolve the division of labor and sharing of competencies that has worked for you up to this point, and even that required frequent fine tuning. Now in a relatively short amount of time you must redefine those role relationships, finding some new sources of personal and shared satisfaction and reshaping some of the old ones. While the changes have an impact on you both, they do so in different ways. Therefore, we will discuss the role change issues for women and for partners separately. We encourage you to read the entire section as an opportunity to gain added insight into your partner's experience.

Compelled to lie down, the woman in premature labor is only too aware of the many roles she used to fulfill. Errand-runner. Wage earner. Gardener. Tennis partner. Lover. Career woman. Dog walker. Cook. Electrician. Hostess. Guest. Now those roles that provided both intrinsic gratification and appreciation from others have been taken away or drastically altered by prescribed bedrest. The loss is undeniable, abated only partially by its temporary nature. To stem the disappointment of the loss, it is important to assess which aspects of each supplanted role were the most important and then to try to regain, through modified or substituted roles, as much as is possible of the lost sense of meaning and productivity.

Whether they had been working outside the home or not, almost all women suddenly confined to bed feel unproductive in relation to their usual standards for a day's accomplishments. You may indeed have found ways to bring the office to you, or to manage the household from your perch. Still, at times you can't get to needed resources as easily as you used to, and your rather fragile physical and emotional condition slows you down. If you're a career woman, you may experience fears that an earlier-than-planned work sabbatical will threaten advancement, keep you out of "circulation" too long, or even jeopardize your job itself. If you're used to being active in the home and community, turning over household tasks to someone else or not seeing them accomplished as you would have can be greatly frustrating.

In addition to work roles, we all occupy socio-emotional roles in relation to those around us. You may have been the social organizer for your family or group of friends. You may have been playmate for your partner, child, or pet. You may have been the confidante of those close to you. You may, indeed, not be able to fulfill some of these roles in ways you did previously. And, in fact, loved ones may turn from you to others, not wanting to impose at this time. This, of course, further reduces the ways in which you feel useful. Watching your partner take on new and added roles while you give them up may make you feel guilty and withdraw further, seeing a predominance of "I can't do's" over "I can do's." From such a posture you may find yourself giving up still more of the ways in which you can be active.

At the same time, you will, indeed, experience periods when you see clearly what you *could* be doing to be more productive, and that's the last thing you *want* to be doing. You have enough to deal with just staying quiet and calm without thinking about what needs to be done or how you could be helpful. Many women report that their time in bed was one of intense self-absorption—a time when they felt disinclined or even unwilling to try to do some of the things they previously did, no matter how possible those things might be. This is true especially early in the confinement period when it requires a lot of energy just to embrace a new position in life. In fact, a moderate shift toward inner reflectiveness can be of great help in coping with the demands of bedrest.

Self-absorption may sound absolutely luxurious to the partner of a woman in premature labor. Frequently, that's just the problem. With the taking on of new roles and tasks come two primary challenges for the partner. One, of course, is to get it all done. Whereas before you may have done your share of the errand-running, household chores, wage earning, shopping, pet and/or child care, now you may have it all to do yourself. At least you have the sole responsibility for picking up what someone else forgot. You probably have increased financial concerns and responsibilities too, changing your relationship to your work in some ways. Your career may, on the one hand, provide some familiar relief from your intensified responsibilities at home. On the other hand, fatigue, preoccupations, and pressures (both practical and financial) may lessen your ability to perform as usual. In addition, you probably feel the desire and the pressure to be an available source of encouragement, entertainment, and understanding for your partner. The directions in which you are torn are many. Role overload can result in decreased performance on all fronts, making it hard to feel like your usual effective self. Most partners cope with this by letting some things slide. Indeed, you have to. Making conscious choices about which things will receive less attention is usually a more effective route than is plunging ahead on all fronts until something breaks—perhaps in the area you least want it to.

That suggests the second challenge of taking on new roles. It is important not to give up all the ways in which you take time for yourself. Be it reading, physical exercise, movies, meditation, or long drives or walks, it is critical to set aside some private time away from work, chores, and partner. You need the time to let things run through your mind, time to reflect on your feelings, time to sort priorities, time to have fun. It is not uncommon for partners to feel guilty when they allow themselves such "luxuries," particularly in light of their mate's restriction to bed. You may even assume that your partner would resent your taking time to yourself— an assumption you may want to check out. It is important to keep in mind that, to the extent that you are able to rejuvenate yourself, you bring fresh energy to your interaction with your partner. In the end, both of you will be better for it.

Coping with Changes
in Your Usual Life Roles

Both of you want to feel useful, effective, wanted and needed. Examine what those words mean for you. For both of you this involves some self-examination, sorting out what aspects of your personalities and capabilities feel central to your self-definition and to your relationship. These underlying elements are the ones that require a central place in your new role divisions. For the woman in premature labor this requires adjusting to some losses and redirecting other needs. For her partner it requires clarifying priorities and letting some things go.

What were the satisfactions in managing and executing household affairs? A sense of order and efficiency? Physical activity? Contact with neighbors and community members? Exercise of your creative talents? A feeling of taking care of your loved ones? What were the payoffs in going to the office? Salary? Contact with co-workers? Enjoyment of the job itself? A sense that you're building your career toward the future?

When "lost" activities are looked at in this light as a composite of rewards, women report that it is easier to see which aspects must indeed be altered or redefined, and which can be accomplished by different means—hence are not lost. Perhaps physical activity must be foregone along with income, but there may be ways to be creative, to organize tasks for others to execute with maximal efficiency for them, to be in contact with neighbors and co-workers, to build your future career, or to take care of those you love from your bed. Take stock of what is really essential for you to feel that you are able to be yourself, mourn what is temporarily lost, and try to recapture as much as possible.

In the latter regard, it is important not to infantilize yourself or let yourself be treated like a child. There are certainly times when being "unproductive" is the most productive thing you can do, times when you just need to be taken care of to replenish the stores of caretaking you're giving to your baby. But while you need support, you also need to be able to support. You need outlets to balance your needs for self-absorption with your ability to consider others. Your partner especially needs encouragement and understanding, and you know better than anyone what many of the tasks, issues, and needs are. Your partner may even be one who would like to protect you from certain worries, such as financial concerns. By insisting that as many areas as possible be open to joint decision-making, the two of you remain a team. You may even take on the research and planning role, directing the execution—at least for a time succumbing to a "brains" versus "brawn" role division in your relationship.

We have already suggested some of the ways that partners might cope with increased duties; i.e., setting priorities, insuring private time. The most obvious remedy for partners, of course, is help. Where and how to get it may seem less obvious. In the best of worlds, at least one of you would have a parent or other relative living close by who could take over many of the household tasks. Many couples ask a parent to live with them temporarily. If you have an available parent with whom you are compatible, and the sacrifice to your privacy is acceptable to you, consider this option seriously. Do, however, consider it carefully before you act. An additional person in the house at this time with whom you have interpersonal difficulties may be more of a burden than dirty dishes. If neither of your families lives close by, perhaps someone could visit for a week. A week's help in stocking the freezer with cooked foods and the pantry with dry goods can last a long time. If you can possibly afford household help, either regularly or occasionally, to clean, shop, or cook, the expenditure will be well worth it. College or high school students are frequently eager to do odds and ends as needed for relatively little money.

As we have suggested above, you and your partner may be able to forge a new brand of teamwork. From her bed, she can plan menus and shopping lists, pay bills, collect information over the phone to minimize your errand or shopping time. Likewise if you have helpers, she can delegate responsibilities. She can't, however, know what is going on in the rest of the house (if for instance you're out of laundry detergent), so you will have to evolve some means of communicating and coordinating. It will take time, but with some humor and a few slip-ups (like no toilet paper for her 2:00 A.M. bathroom stop) you will work it out with surprising efficiency.

Finally, some hints on what to say when genuinely interested friends and family ask what they can do to help. Please *do* tell them something.

— Cook an extra batch of their favorite recipe with which you can stock your freezer. (Wrapped in serving portions is even better.)

— Pick up the prescription or dry cleaning on their way over to visit.

— Lend you some board games for a change of pace.

— Join a painting party to paint or wallpaper the nursery.

— Take your other children for the afternoon.

— Take over a regular chore, such as picking up the kids from school or mowing the lawn.

As a couple you want again to feel that you are each holding up your end of the deal. How you work out the specifics will depend on your individual and joint talents, interests, and styles. Extending your pregnancy has become your major goal, and you each are doing your respective parts. You are indeed a team in this effort, with both of your roles absolutely essential.

JOE'S STORY

My wife, Laura, was gradually put on complete bedrest over a period of a month. At twenty-six weeks of gestation, I was left entirely in charge of the household. I took our son, Aaron, to his toddler group once a week. I was usually the only father there. The other mothers would praise me for all I was doing to keep the normal systems running at home—food, childcare, etc. I told them that I felt that I had the easy job—I had a day's worth of accomplishments to look back on. All my wife had at the end of each day was the relief that she hadn't gone into labor, while trying to maintain some sense of self-worth beyond being a "birth machine." The disruption of our normal lives and routines was complete. We'd go to bed at night not knowing whether we'd end up in the hospital by morning. No news was good news. One night we ended up in a labor room of the hospital where, two years earlier, our son had been born. I hadn't been there since the night of that miracle. I felt turned inside out by the emotions of being there, hearing babies being born down the hall, trying desperately to hold back, to halt this skid towards premature birth that we seemed to have no control over. Luckily, we were able to "hold on" to our pregnancy that night, and were discharged home to bedrest the next morning.

After the initial weeks of "taking over" the house, I slowly tried to integrate my professional work (writer) into this routine. I didn't have the lengthy stretches of time I was used to, but I'd grab a few hours before my son would awaken, or during naps. As if by perfect design, I was currently working on a rewrite job of a script about a woman who was trying to do it all—family, job, community—and running herself into the ground. I identified totally and found solace in the darkest hours of my own struggle, believing that these experiences in my own life would surely "inform" my writing. Just like the woman, I was determined to be the provider, the nurturer, the companion. As my deadline approached, I slowly realized that the script wasn't getting written. I got an extension and blew that too. I had failed to grasp how totally the ordeal of what we were going through had depleted my resources. I had nothing left for the writing. Finally, I returned the script and the advance money I'd been given to the producer with my apologies. As I drove home, the impact of what I'd done hit me—all those days and nights of putting my family ahead of my work had led to this. I had never seriously considered that I couldn't pull it all off. I felt isolated, like a failure, as I drove home hopefully to make it through another day.

When we reached thirty-eight weeks, our doctor told us it was okay to have the baby. Instead of feeling relief, my reaction was to go into a block-buster depression. Finally one night I spewed out to my wife about how much I felt I'd had to give up, how angry I was with all we'd had to put up with, and above all, the feeling that somehow we were being punished with what we'd had to go through with this baby. I could feel all the fears and resentments I'd been sitting on for all those weeks finally rising to the surface. Now I could let it out without the fear that it might set off another run of contractions. Eventually the darkness passed as I began for the first time to look forward to the birth.

The night our daughter was born, I was carrying her out of the labor room down the hall to the nursery and my eyes met those of a man who was standing in the hall, clearly an "expectant father." He congratulated me and I asked him if his wife was about to deliver. He pointed to a room and said his wife was in there at twenty-two weeks, on Ritodrine. How my heart went out to him. I tried to give him some words of consolation or encouragement, to hold up my baby so he could see what it was that he would be fighting to protect in the weeks to come. But the difference between us was so obvious—I had my baby, and he had sixteen weeks to go.

> *Joe Landon, father of Aaron (two years)
> and Emily (three months).*

FINANCIAL CHANGES

Bedrest may signal an earlier-than-planned loss of the woman's contribution to the family income. It certainly will mean increased costs in medical bills, supplies, and services. When these factors add strain to an already tight budget, financial worries can form a backdrop of tension for your family life. Many couples find this a difficult area to talk about, especially at this time. You may feel that you have no choice but to spend the necessary money. You may even feel twinges of guilt for even thinking about money "at a time like this," and so try to push the worries from your mind.

Avoidance of money issues may arise for both of you from a wish to protect the other. Many women report that they don't want their partners to feel that they're questioning whether all their partner's hard work will provide enough. From such a point of view, raising these issues may feel like a vote of no confidence at a time when that's the last thing you want to suggest. Where money's concerned it's tempting to feel that if you're not contributing tangibly, you should not contribute verbally either, and therefore should say nothing. For the partner, the avoidance of money issues may stem from feeling pressured to "provide." You now have so much responsibility that it can be easy to assume you have it all. You may especially not want to worry your partner. Avoidance of money issues, however, can only divide you as a couple and allow fearful fantasies to grow.

At the other end of the continuum from avoidance of money issues is preoccupation with them. For some, worry about money can replace worry about the baby. Money is, after all, much more tangible and potentially more controllable. It can become another means by which you "try to be good," to insure a happy ending. That is, the metaphor of trying to cut out all that isn't necessary (as the woman may have to do physically) can be applied to your finances as well. But all that accomplishes, in many cases, is to leave you feeling deprived yet again.

Finances are a challenge for most couples to handle. Financial strain is, indeed, a leading cause of marital discord. You no doubt are familiar with the flavor of your usual disagreements about money. This will in all probability determine how money affects you now, with greater intensity depending upon the degree of strain. With some reflection, this time can pose an opportunity for you to resolve some differences, as suggested below.

Coping with Financial Changes

From the foregoing discussion it is clear that we are advancing two bits of advice. The first, of course, is that you in some way share your financial concerns at this time. That may mean discussing which bills to postpone, whether to take out a loan, which items in your budget to forego. It may mean agreeing that one of you is indeed more able or willing than the other to deal with money right now. Whatever is the most comfortable mode for you of dealing with money matters, we recommend that it be made explicit so that money doesn't become a ghost in your closet.

For many couples, money is frequently a symbol or metaphor for an aspect of their relationship. Thus it can become an arena for working out other issues. Interactions about money may mirror how you handle decision-making in general, how the two of you feel about control versus risk, how you express joy and caution. Concerns about money now, in addition to their reality in and of themselves, may represent other feelings as well. Exploring money as a symbol for each of you may help in getting past an impasse, should one arise.

The second bit of advice is not to cut out all the luxuries. You need a few special surprises to take the edge off your deprivation and to help you each feel appreciated. Just as mobile pregnant women are advised to buy a new dress in the last trimester to pick up their spirits, a new nightgown or two can go a long way toward raising yours. Likewise, partners need to indulge themselves from time to time as a reward and a relief.

A number of other practical steps have been passed on to us by women in premature labor. They include the following:

— Check your insurance policies. Premature labor is a complication of pregnancy covered up to 80 percent of allowable costs by most medical insurance policies. Generally there is a maximum amount of costs to you, the insured, after which the insurance company will pay 100 percent. Often insurance companies cover the cost of medications. Inquire into this, as the medication costs for premature labor can be quite high. Also check your plan's coverage of newborn infants, to be sure the first thirty days of life are not excluded.

— Talk with your employer about the type of disability plan under which you are covered and request the necessary forms. Although the amount of disability income is often less than your actual income was, it does not usually qualify as taxable income.

FEELINGS OF DEPENDENCY
AND POWERLESSNESS

There were times when I'd feel especially inspired to do some writing. John would bring me books and paper before he left. I'd enthusiastically begin, only to have a brilliant idea that required the file in the next room. Then I was torn between risking an extra trip and feeling defeated. Over the about six trillion occasions in which this

*type of situation arose, I chose between those two options
about an equal number of times.*

Expectant Mother

Dependency and powerlessness (or lack of control) are two of the most frequent complaints about confinement to bed during premature labor. While particularly acute for the woman in bed, her partner frequently experiences parallel feelings of powerlessness. For both, being subject to a physical process about which medicine knows relatively little, taxes the usual "take charge" coping mechanisms. We will discuss each in turn.

A woman's sudden inability to get or do for herself can be frustrating, maddening, and depressing. While this is true in itself, other factors can help or hinder her ability to accept the real need to depend upon others while confined to bed.

Asking others to help does not come easily to those of us reared in the mainstream of our culture's Judeo-Christian traditions. We are implicitly taught that it is better to give than to receive, to suffer than to impose. It is especially difficult to do so when you feel as if you can't return the favor, and yet you need it so much. There are probably one or two "safe" people to ask—your partner, a friend or relative, someone you pay a wage to be helpful. But after a while you may feel badly about all your asking and want either to spread your requests around or to stop asking altogether. The latter solution, of course, invites further problems in that you lose more control over your situation. It is only by asking others to help that you can remain active and involved.

One recently advanced theory of depression[2] holds that depressed individuals have been in situations where they have learned through repeated incidents that they are helpless to control a painful outcome. This "learned helplessness" phenomenon can certainly apply to the woman confined to bed and her partner if repeated efforts to marshal materials and resources either fail or lead to other negative consequences (such as feeling that you're a burden). It also can be applied to the situation where contractions or cervical changes continue to occur despite the best efforts of both of you to follow the prescribed treatment.

You both need to feel as though what you do makes a difference, as though you have some control over your circumstances. This requires

---

2. Seligman, M. E. P. Depression and learned helplessness. In *The Psychology of Depression: Contemporary Theory and Research*, ed. R. J. Friedman and M. M. Katz. New York: John Wiley and Sons, 1974, pp. 83–113.

some assertion and taking of control; however, there are some built-in elements to the premature labor experience that may make assertion and control difficult. Recognizing them may help you to address them.

The woman in bed may encounter pressures and expectations that come from being in the "patient role." You are flat on your back. Ordinarily someone in your position is sick. You are not; but your position invites others to see you in the sick role. Medical sociologists have talked about the patient role as one in which the patient is seen as "not responsible" but rather, as a victim of the body. "The body" is then given up to "the experts" for fixing. What results is, of course, depersonalization of the individuals. Some women in premature labor report that medical personnel, rather than talking to them about their condition, talk past them to their partner. There can be a tendency among family and friends to be "protective" as well, seeing you as the fragile sick person and thus enhancing your dependency.

Earlier (while discussing worry about the baby) we alluded to the lack of control frequently felt by partners of women in premature labor. As helpless as she may feel, the woman at least can do some things to directly affect the pregnancy, such as staying in bed, taking medications, etc. You, the partner, on the other hand, have an important but indirect impact on the course of events. You may find yourself monitoring your partner's compliance in taking pills and staying horizontal, even getting angry over an extra trip or forgotten pill here and there. This, of course, is an attempt to assert more direct control. Other ways in which you may seek some control are through information and through managing your partner's care. Both are important ways in which you do influence a successful outcome. Your work and support are essential to your partner's ability to comply with the necessary treatment, and to do so with some sanity.

If your experience involves hospitalization you will no doubt recognize many elements that can promote feelings of dependency and powerlessness in both of you. In a hospital it is difficult to feel that you have control over your time or your privacy. The helpful staff there will recognize your need to do so. Seek them out. Likewise, sensitive practitioners will recognize your right and your wish to be continuously informed and involved regarding your treatment. There are things that you can do to affect the situation both for your own sense of involvement and for the welfare of your baby.

Coping with Feelings of
Dependency and Powerlessness

Feelings of helplessness and dependency can be experienced as vague and all-encompassing. However, such feelings do not come out of thin air. They are tied to reality (which may sometimes be modified) or to interpretations of reality (which may also, and perhaps more easily, be modified). Recognizing the sources of feelings of futility and helplessness can be a first step to taking control. Ask others to deal with you directly; be assertive in getting medical information. Chapter Six offers some suggestions for gaining a sense of control while you are hospitalized.

At home you have more control over your routine; so much so, in fact, that you may feel as if there is no routine. Many women remark that creating one is helpful for feeling in control of the passage of time. You will find ways to have at your fingertips the materials you need to carry out your routines. Make lists of things you need and feel free to curse when you forget to include an item. Create options for how to spend a particular period of time so that if one alternative is blocked you don't feel stuck. Chapter Five provides more hints for establishing routines and managing space.

Those who subscribe to the "learned helplessness" theory of depression make two points about it. When one accepts helplessness one usually assumes a passive position, refusing to continue efforts to gain control. One may thus be unaware that circumstances have changed. For example, if your early experience is that your amount of immobility has little effect on your contractions, you may decide that you have no impact, and thus feel a sense of futility throughout your experience. The truth may be that indeed your inactivity is important, but that the initial overriding influence was the electrochemical process already in motion. Once controlled by drugs, your activity level may take over as the predominant factor. If, however, you resign yourself to feelings of futility, you may deprive yourself of this realization and of the consequent feelings of effectiveness.

What this implies is that how you interpret the situation and what you say to yourself about it can be of major importance. If you assume that asking is imposing, then indeed you won't ask. If you assume that your medical caregivers will tell you what you need to know, then you will hear only what they presume your interests and concerns to be. However, if you view yourselves as remarkably flexible and as doing the best you can for your baby and yourselves, you will feel and be more powerful.

ANGER

> *I had a dream one night after eight weeks in bed that the
> bed caught on fire. Then the curtains caught and those
> monotonous four walls were consumed. I got out of the
> room and was scared at first. Then I started running
> away. I ran and ran and ran. It felt so good.*
>
>   *Expectant Mother*

> *I come home and she's depressed or bored or into her TV
> show—totally zoned out. She says she has nothing to talk
> about. What about me? Ask me! I have lots to talk
> about! But I sure get tired of hearing "Oh, that's nice."*
>
>   *Expectant Father*

Anger may seem to be either an overwhelming or useless emotion. In
truth, it is an expression of your vitality and involvement. You are neither
dispassionate nor passive. You care about the quality of your life; you care
about your loved ones. Anger is motivated by the wish to protect either
yourself or someone/something about which you care. It is the "fight"
aspect of your primitive "fight/flight" response capability. It is essential to
total well-being.

However, compared to primitive situations, the issues that arouse our
modern "fight/flight" responses are more complex. The threats are more
ambiguous, our possible responses more varied. Over our growing-up years
we learn all sorts of ways to respond to threatening situations—some direct, some indirect; some adaptive, some maladaptive. Yet all are designed
to protect something dear to us. All are designed, in one way or another,
to assert some control.

Premature labor is a situation bound to arouse your need to protect
yourself, your child, your loved ones—and hence, to awaken angry feelings. But it is a situation in which, as we have discussed, control is not
easily taken. You probably expect that when you get angry at someone or
something they or it will change. The need for bedrest won't change as a
result of getting angry, so it can be hard to know where to direct the
anger. Do you yell at the bed? Your doctor? Your cervix?

You are both bound to become angry—sick and tired of the situation.
Here are some ways anger might manifest itself.

General irritability. You may become short-tempered at everything and everyone. Both of you require some semblance of orderliness and predictability in your suddenly restricted and chaotic situation. When things don't go smoothly or on schedule, you don't have the usual reserves to be flexibly tolerant. You may blow up at the pharmacist who doesn't have your prescription in stock. When your co-worker arrives late you may become annoyed at the lack of consideration. Your mother's telephone call may seem like an intrusion. Even the cut flowers brought by the neighbor may feel like only a puny drop in the bucket of your need to be cheered up. All of these incidents are speaking to the larger factors that contribute to your anger. You feel unable to get what you need, unrecognized, intruded upon, and patronized. That is, the incident about which you feel angry may, in actuality, be a symbol for some underlying feelings. Regarding it in this light may help you to see your true feelings more clearly and to express them more directly, as we will discuss below.

Anger at loved ones. Those to whom we feel close are often safe objects for our anger. Whereas you can't take it out on your boss, maybe you can yell at your partner or another loved one. Of course, this is always a phenomenon in intimate relationships, but it may be especially frequent now. Your partner or parent or friend just can't do enough—that's a reality and a frustration. You usually turn to them to make it better. Now it seems that they may be able to make it better, but not enough better. They can't stop the contractions, take away the bills, or ease the boredom.

Conflicts manifested in fights are almost inevitable in such a stressful situation as premature labor, but close relationships can absorb and tolerate them as a necessary means of releasing anger. It is helpful, after the emotional release of such a fight, to reach some understanding of the issues involved. This may include some self-examination and perhaps the recognition that you were really angry with yourself or with the situation. More will be said about this below.

Physical agitation. For the woman confined to bed, anger at immobility may take the obvious form of physical agitation—tics, nervous habits, the urge to hit or kick something. Your body does want some activity, and trying to inhibit it has emotional and physical consequences. Refer to Chapter Nine and speak with your medical practitioner about some safe exercises you might do in bed. It may be that this can alleviate one source of frustration. If you are one for whom physical activity is a way of venting anger, safe exercise may still provide a means of coping at times when you are angry.

Depression. Anger that does not find release can be turned upon oneself, resulting in self-reproach, general malaise, and depression. Expression of anger may be blocked for a number of reasons. Many women fear that unrestrained emotion will trigger another round of contractions. While it is true that intense emotional stress can exacerbate contractions, trying to contain or divert anger can lead to even more emotional stress. It is generally more advisable to express feelings before they escalate.

Both women and their partners sometimes report that they feel guilty in a superstitious way about their angry feelings. You may feel that you should be grateful not to have delivered so far. If you act ungrateful (i.e., get angry), you may be punished. However, it is possible to feel grateful and angry at the same time. Just as brave does not necessarily mean a lack of fear, acceptance of a situation sometimes includes anger. Depression, lethargy, tears, lack of appetite are signals that you may not have acknowledged your anger. We will suggest how to do so below.

Coping with Anger

Several additional considerations about dealing with anger may be made. One involves getting in touch with the sources of your frustration. Another concerns expressing them.

For some people, the expression of anger comes easily and directly. For others it is more inhibited and even hard to detect. If you identified with some of the indirect indications of anger mentioned above, you may want to put some effort into pinpointing what makes you mad.

As suggested above, listening to the symbolic level of what you say or what gets your goat is one way. If you blow up when your favorite TV program is replaced by a special, then the underlying anger may have to do with control over your own time. That is, what was critical in this event was that your attempt to plan your time was thwarted by factors beyond your control. You will be forever unsuccessful in retrieving the TV show, but realizing that the larger issue is control over your time may enable you to exert some power over your time elsewhere. When something piques your anger, take some time to reflect on the issues or factors inherent in the situation. What does the circumstance symbolize or represent? Let yourself give voice to your angry feelings and listen to what comes forth as a way of getting clues to the underlying issues.

Another way to identify sources of anger is simply to make a list: "I am mad at (because) . . ." You may have to force the first couple of answers, but soon words will come to mind fairly easily. Write down whatever comes to mind. There may be categories of things that will give you some insights. The goals here are both to express your feelings and to make them concrete, so that something can be done about them.

Expressing anger constructively to others has been the topic for entire books and workshops. Here we will offer only a few tips.

1. Try to state your feelings in "I" format. That is, instead of "You always . . ." try "I feel . . .". The "you" form tends to put others on the defensive, while "I" tends to invite understanding. It also encourages you to "own" your feelings or be clear about just what it is you feel.

2. Make your complaints as specific and concrete as possible. That is, try "When you said ————— this morning, I felt —————" rather than "You never listen." This may require some reflection beforehand, which in the heat of the moment may be difficult. Nonetheless, it is usually helpful over the course of a disagreement to try to be specific. Again, criticism of a behavior generally makes a person feel less attacked than does criticism of a trait. People generally feel more able and inclined to reconsider specific behavior than they do a general trait.

3. Actively listen to your partner. When possible, try to rephrase what you understand your partner's feelings to be. You can help your partner to clarify and express the source of their anger. This is, of course, easier when you are not the target, but even if you are, understanding can go a long way toward relieving the feeling.

Finally, there may be instances when the issue behind your angry feelings is not control but rather acceptance. Throughout this book we will propose a perspective in which life events can be seen as opportunities for personal learning and growth. One way of unlocking this realm of self-discovery is to listen to the metaphoric level of meaning in significant situations. Let us return to the example of the replacement of a favorite TV program by a special. An examination of this circumstance on a metaphoric level would look at "double meanings" in the words used. In this case, the word "special" comes to mind. Indeed, in premature labor, your entire normal schedule has been cancelled and replaced by "special" circumstances. The TV incident reflects, in microcosm, the larger life situation, and thus arouses feelings. The next step is to reflect upon the challenge presented. This will have personal relevance, and in this situation might range from simple acknowledgement that things can't be as they were to a deeper acceptance and appreciation of the value of the "special." The challenge is to embrace the new "show" and to see what it has to offer.

CHANGES IN SEXUAL RELATIONS

In this area, your obstetric practitioner may have recommended anything from completely curbing all sexual activity involving vaginal penetration or leading to orgasm, to no restrictions at all. But even if you have been given no medical restrictions on sex, you may both feel rather cautious about rocking the boat, so to speak. For many couples, sexual intimacy is a vital part of the relationship. Limitations in this area may appear to block yet another avenue toward closeness.

All in all, we know very little at this point about how and to what extent premature labor brings about changes in sexual expression. That it does change is an assumption we make based on (1) the treatment generally recommended by medical personnel and (2) the sometimes joking complaints made by patients. Specific concerns with regard to sexual activity as it relates to premature labor include (1) the possible stimulation of uterine contractions by orgasm and/or by the action of the prostaglandin chemical found in the semen of the male partner, and (2) possible infection caused by bacteria transmitted in intercourse, especially if there is a cervical cerclage in place. However, not enough research has been done to provide specific guidelines for sexual activity for most couples with premature labor. Some clinicians suggest the use of a condom with intercourse to prevent the exposure of the cervix to prostaglandins from the semen. Other practitioners recommend no intercourse at all (e.g., in a case of placenta previa). Ask your clinician at various points in your pregnancy about sexual activity; some form of sexual activity may be acceptable at thirty-four weeks of pregnancy but not at twenty-eight weeks. A variety of factors may be involved in the recommendation. We hope to gain further knowledge of how premature labor affects sexual activity and vice versa, as more research is done on this question.

We do know some things about sexual activity during pregnancy in general. Briefly, the frequency of sexual intercourse for most couples does not appear to decline in the second trimester, but does do so increasingly in each month of the third trimester. The frequency of female orgasm does appear to decline during the second and third trimesters, and is closely associated with the level of sexual interest on the part of the woman. Preferred positions shift as pregnancy progresses, from male superior to female superior, side to side, and rear entry positions. Many couples prefer to practice mutual masturbation during the last month. These trends, of course, describe couples in general; the variety of ways in which particular couples enjoy sex during pregnancy is virtually limitless.

Anecdotal reports from couples experiencing premature labor suggest that by and large they follow the same pattern of declining female desire for sex and the use of alternate modes of sexual expression. Some women report that they try to abstain from orgasm themselves, but continue to pleasure their partners through touch, masturbation, and oral-genital sex. Some women appear to enjoy fondling and cuddling. Other women seem to find caressing too stimulating and frustrating, preferring to refrain.

One or both of you may find that you don't desire sex as you used to. It may help to remember that this is common for women late in pregnancy even without the complications of premature labor. Other factors that may affect sexual desire include fatigue, physical discomfort, feelings of unattractiveness, and fears about the effects of arousal on contractions. Female orgasms *can* stimulate contractions, so follow your clinician's advice in this regard. Breast stimulation, either with early nipple preparation for breastfeeding, or within a sexual context, can cause uterine contractions. Breast stimulation should be avoided in women with premature labor until thirty-seven weeks of gestation. What may happen, however, is that the fear of orgasm can generalize to a fear of arousal, and lead further to avoidance of physical intimacy altogether. Thus, as a means of self-protection you may find yourselves feeling numb to any sexual desire at all.

On the other hand, sexual restrictions may leave you with tremendous unsated desires. You may find yourself having arousing dreams that may even lead to orgasm. It is important to recognize sexual frustration as such and to talk about it with your partner. It can easily be displaced onto other areas, leading to arguments about otherwise inconsequential things or exacerbating other problems. Giving a name to your frustration can at least help you to feel desired by the other and make you partners in creative intimacy.

Coping with Changes in Sexual Relations

While we urge you to follow your obstetric practitioner's advice and your own intuition where sex is concerned, we also urge you not to close off all doors to physical affection. This includes, of course, not cutting off communication about it. Share with your partner what you would like, what he or she does that makes you feel good, how you feel about the limitations you may have on sexual relations. Sexuality for most people is a highly sensitive area, often difficult to talk about openly.

The changes in your familiar habits of relating sexually may give rise to fearful fantasies about your partner's feelings or thoughts. Such fanta-

sies can only serve to increase your sexual distance from one another. If
you have such fantasies, check them out. When doing so we recommend
these simple guidelines.

1. The discloser should *state* the fantasy as a fantasy, e.g., "I have a
fantasy (or I imagine) that you are turned off to me sexually."

2. The responder should *validate* or acknowledge any aspect of the
fantasy that is true, e.g., "It is true that I haven't initiated sex and that
I'm scared to get aroused."

3. The responder should *correct* any misperceptions in the fantasy,
e.g., "I do find you arousing; I am just closed down sexually in general
because I'm afraid to get excited."

The two of you can then together explore what you may want to do
to change the situation.

There are ways to explore physical affection without necessarily stimulating genital arousal. Cuddling and kissing can help to satisfy the need
for touching, while also communicating much-needed encouragement, appreciation, and love. Indeed, touch can produce pleasure without necessarily leading to sexual relations. Your circumstances may provide you an
opportunity to discover some new sensuous experiences.

One means of nongenital touching is through what are referred to as
sensate focus exercises. They are so called because they attempt to focus a
couple's attention on a wider range of sensations than genital arousal
alone. We include two as alternatives for sharing physically intimate time
together.[3]

1. Give one another a mini-massage. Pick an area far from your
genitals that would give you pleasure, e.g., your hand, foot, face, head.
One difference in this approach is that the person giving the massage
should focus on what feels good to do, not on what might please the
receiver. Thus the massager will reappreciate the pleasures that touching,
in and of itself, can have. The recipient need do nothing but relax and
enjoy. Then switch roles.

2. Explore nongenital body parts using different textures and materials. Again, alternate the roles of giving and receiving. Collect a number of

[3] Adapted from Barbach, Lonnie G. *For Yourself: The Fulfillment of Female
Sexuality.* Garden City, N.Y.: Anchor Press/Doubleday, 1976.

materials—feathers, satin, wool, oil, brushes, etc. Use them to explore your partner's body. Again, the giver should concentrate primarily on what feels good to do and only secondarily on the receiver's pleasure. Feel the diffcrent textures against your partner's body. Switch roles.

You may invent additional ways to spend nongenital touching time. During premature labor the woman's body receives much clinical attention and her partner's body perhaps little attention at all. It can be important to try to reembrace your physical, affectionate selves, to repersonalize and resexualize in some form your bodies and your relationship.

LOSS OF THE FANTASIZED PREGNANCY

> *When our obstetrician told us we couldn't use the Alternative Birthing Room because we were at higher risk for complications of labor—that did it. It seemed like we already had to give up so much, and now we couldn't even look forward to that.*
>
> *Expectant Mother*

You probably have had some images of how it would be to be pregnant parents. You may have imagined enjoying the last few months of being together as a couple, perhaps a vacation, long walks, or romantic dinners. Your fantasy probably included preparing for the baby—decorating a nursery, shopping for clothes and accessories. Before becoming bedridden you may have enjoyed all the attention that pregnancy attracts in public and from friends and family. If you already have children, you probably imagined more time with them in their active worlds.

This imagined pregnancy experience is lost to you. As with any loss, you are probably experiencing aspects of the mourning process. Of course, this mourning is not as acute as when a loved one is lost. Nonetheless, there are some feelings shared by couples in premature labor that seem to be better understood when recognized as feelings of loss.

You may find yourselves tending to avoid your still-active pregnant friends. You may not be able to prevent yourself from feeling somewhat resentful of and/or even inadequate in relation to them. Negative feelings directed toward friends are hard to acknowledge to yourself. Doing so, however, may clarify your feelings of sadness at not being able to do as much as they can. In this way you deal with the real feelings that your avoidance represents.

Some obstetric practitioners feel that, to be safe, couples who have experienced premature labor should ultimately deliver under fully equipped medical conditions, ruling out the use of an Alternative Birth Center (ABC). If your practitioner is one who feels this way and you were counting on an ABC birth, you may be quite upset at the loss. Currently there is much in the media to make such births sound appealing and romantic. Indeed, there is a lot to be said for a homey atmosphere, your partner's presence, and an early checkout. One negative aspect of the current movement toward alternative births is that, indeed, it can become a pressure to have the "perfect" birth. Those who don't experience unmedicated, vaginal deliveries in a birthing room or at home may feel like a "failure" in comparison to the modern "ideal." We seem to have lost sight of the "alternative" concept, and to have created a new norm. The fact is that about 50 percent of couples intending to use an ABC eventually do not do so, for one reason or another. Many couples report that, in the intensity of labor, what they thought would be important isn't; the baby's health and mother's comfort loom larger.

Each birth, no matter what the surroundings, is a special event. Even if the Alternative Birth Center is not used, the birth can still be a personal and fulfilling event. When a birth takes place in a labor room, the mother can often breastfeed immediately and integrate other parts of a planned ABC birth. Even if birth is by Cesarean section, a LeBoyer bath may be available for the baby in the recovery room, breastfeeding can be fairly immediate (usually within a half hour), and the family will be able to be together for a few hours. If a private room can be arranged, the other parent may be able to "room in" along with the baby. The challenge to you is to create your own alternative for birthing and with an open mind, to work toward a birth that is "perfect" for the needs of you and your baby.

Some parents find that they begin to feel cautious about imagining the fetus and fantasizing what it will be like to be parents. Of course, this withdrawal is self-protective. Your pregnancy has suffered a threat and you do what you can to avoid further hurt. While some of this is to be expected, it may also be in part an overgeneralization of your mourning of the fantasized pregnancy. You have not lost your child; you have lost mobility during pregnancy. You may feel less lonely and more purposeful if you can mourn your lost experience, but recognize what is still present— your connection to your growing baby.

Coping with Feelings of Loss

The grieving process commonly includes a number of aspects that may be applied in a general way to your feelings of loss. The first common aspect of grief is denial. You may at first have minimized the impact that inactivity would have, telling yourselves that it will be only temporary, will mean only slight changes. Denial will at some point give way to recognition of your loss and feelings of sadness at not being able to enact your fantasies. Anger is a typical accompaniment to this sadness. Questioning is an aspect of grief that is somewhat related to anger. You may ask: "Why us?" "What did we do to end up here?" "If we do something or learn something, can we change it?" Sadness and anger are not likely to be one-time feelings. They may recur over time and in different contexts. Sadness may even surface or resurface after your child is born, or even a year later in an "anniversary reaction" to your bed experience. It is almost as though you can feel sympathy for your experience from a distance, whereas while you were in it your energy went wholly into coping. Finally, one comes by degrees to achieve genuine acceptance of the circumstances. You are able to proceed with your reality, having acknowledged the loss and perhaps ascribed some meaning or purpose to the situation. You may then be better able to see the opportunities and alternatives inherent in it.

As time progresses in your pregnancy and you begin to feel more confident about its outcome, you will probably find that your images of the baby and yourselves as parents reemerge. We encourage you to enjoy these growing feelings of attachment as a means both of preparing to have a child and of creating closeness with your baby now. Such closeness now will help you to feel like a family already working toward a common goal. You may have more quiet time together than does a mobile pregnant couple. This time provides an opportunity for you to tune in to your baby and to share this precious time as a family. Chapter Ten suggests some visualization exercises that you may want to try.

SARA'S STORY*

Sitting in the obstetrician's waiting room on a sunny April morning, I marvel at my fortune. I feel I have sneaked in under the wire—getting married for

---

* We are grateful to *Esquire Magazine* for the permission to reprint this portion of "Having It All" by Sara Davidson (June 1984).

the second time at thirty-eight and having a baby at thirty-nine. Across from me are two women with very young babies. I discover that they both had to stay in bed for most of their pregnancies. A chill runs through me. "You couldn't get up, not even to eat? That's horrible."

My husband reaches for my hand. "Don't worry," he says with his wonderful optimism, "it won't happen to you."

Ha.

One of the things people don't tell you about having a baby late in life is that the chances of having trouble carrying the baby are greatly increased.

I was in excellent health when I became pregnant, and I expected to jog and work up to the last day. In a routine visit during my fourth month, the doctor said I appeared to be having problems. I would have to lie on my back with my hips elevated for the rest of my term, or the force of gravity might bring the baby out prematurely.

I was incredulous. I felt fine, and I could not believe anything was seriously wrong. So I cheated. I got out of bed, first for one thing, then for another, until I was walking about more than half the day. During my sixth month I went in for a checkup and was sent straight to the hospital in premature labor.

They strapped a fetal monitor around my stomach, put my head down and my feet up, and pumped me full of intravenous drugs to stop the contractions. The drugs made my heart race 120 beats per minute. My neck was pulsing, my gums, fingers, stomach—everything had the rapid hammer beat. I was short of breath, sweating; the sheets came off steaming, as if from an iron.

From the rooms on either side I could hear women screaming, "It hurts, oh God, my insides are coming out! Heeeellp!" They were delivering babies, but I thought I was in the Gulag, hearing the other prisoners being tortured.

What had happened? I had walked into the hospital looking radiant in a Laura Ashley dress, and now I was weak, panting for breath, with sheet burns on my back and bruises on my arms from the IV. I wanted to pull out the tubes and rip off the belts and run out of the hospital, and just as I was cracking, one of the nurses brought in a tiny baby from the nursery.

"This is what you're working for," she said.

I was startled. I had forgotten I was pregnant.

After this my husband virtually moved into the hospital to keep my spirits up. He brought in our stereo and video recorder and meals from restaurants. When he did go home, he would call and play the piano and sing Cole Porter songs. "Birds do it, bees do it . . ."

Together we managed to weather it out until my condition had stabilized and I could go home. Everyone told me, "As soon as the baby comes, you'll forget the pain." Not a chance, I thought, I won't forget this.

But I did. At this moment I am pregnant with our second child, lying on a rented hospital bed with my hips up and a word processor positioned over my stomach. This time I am not cheating.

> Sara Davidson, mother of
> Andrew (three years) and
> Rachel (five months).

STRESS: YOUR BODY'S RESPONSE; YOUR PSYCHE'S RESPONSE

Thus far, we have presented some common challenges that are likely to affect all couples who experience premature labor to one degree or another. As we noted earlier, each individual and couple will also be faced with challenges unique to them—challenges that arise because of individual circumstances and personalities. In order to solve the problems of such situations, it is helpful to have a framework for how stress occurs and how resolutions to stressful circumstances are achieved.

One cannot talk about stress without reference to the mind-body relationship. We generally think of stress as an external phenomenon—something that happens *to* us. In actuality, stress is at once a stimulus and a response. A stressful situation begins with an event that is perceived by the individual as threatening. Some events are more or less universally perceived as threatening, e.g., fire, violence, serious illness. Other events are threatening only for some, e.g., public speaking, social occasions, high places. Still other events are unique in their threat to only one individual, e.g., an offhand comment that pushed a sensitive button. The first requirement for something to be stressful is for it to be *perceived* as a threat. The mind and the senses interact to initiate a stress response.

The "fight/flight" response is a universal, primal mechanism for responding to threats and challenges. A perceived stressor triggers the body to mobilize resources for either confrontation or escape. Hormones and neurochemicals are released providing extra energy and alertness. *It is this mobilization of body resources to meet a threat that is stress.* Defined this way, stress is neither positive nor negative. It is not something done to us. Rather, stress is a very useful mobilization of energy and resources that we achieve to cope with challenges. Without stress we would be missing an important spur to accomplishment.

All this energy must find an outlet. That is, stress is not only a response to a threatening event, but also a stimulus to action. However, in many modern situations neither fight nor flight is appropriate. When the boss criticizes our work, it may not be wise either to attack or to walk out of the room. Threatened with premature delivery of your baby, you can neither argue your way out of it nor run away. The outlets are less clearly defined. Thus, in modern times we witness increased indicators of mismanaged stress (e.g., irritability, fatigue, sleeplessness, illness, generalized anxiety and tension).

One does do something with stress; one uses it to fuel coping responses, and a coping response can be either effective or ineffective. We all, over time, settle on familiar coping strategies to handle our familiar stresses; for example, when Uncle Ralph tells you for the sixteen-billionth time that if you'd gone into micro computers you'd be on easy street by now, you turn a deaf ear, reminding yourself of how much you enjoy your work and how your financial situation is comfortable enough, thank you. You funnel the energy of your irritation into bolstering your own goals and self-esteem. In times of crisis, however, your usual coping responses may fail. If things aren't going so well at work and finances are tight, Uncle Ralph's remark may put you over the edge. Your old self-talk fails and his remark hits a new sore spot; you can no longer ignore him. An alternative coping strategy is needed.

We can speak of this situation of failed coping as both a danger and an opportunity.[4] There is the danger that the alternative coping employed may be less adaptive in the long run, leading to further problems. For example, you could either erupt at Uncle Ralph or take his criticisms to heart, becoming depressed and immobilized over your poor past decision. On the other hand, a new coping response may be more adaptive, leading to better circumstances. You could use the opportunity to let Uncle Ralph know how his unhelpful remarks make you feel, perhaps forging a better relationship, or you could use the catalyst to productively examine your work situation and make some changes.

Premature labor presents you with many stressful events, both as individuals and as a couple. Your familiar means of channeling stress may be unavailable to you. You may not be able to turn to work or exercise as a source of self-esteem or energy release. You may not have the extra funds to pay for stress relief such as takeout food or household help. You need new coping strategies, hopefully more adaptive ones. Whenever possible you'll want to embrace the opportunity in the situation and avoid the dangers.

---

[4] Morley, W. E. Theory of crisis intervention. *Pastoral Psychology*, April, 1970.

We have attempted in the first part of the chapter to outline some coping alternatives for the common stressors of premature labor. Now we offer you a framework for analyzing your more individual stressors. Please refer to the worksheet at the end of the chapter. We include three: one for each of you individually, and one for you to use as a couple. The first column invites you to list the event or stressor. This may be anything from a particularly painful interaction with someone to a major personal loss, anything that puts you over the edge, leaving you at a loss for what to do. The more specific you are, the better. Try to get at just what was the "straw that broke the camel's back." It was that sentence in Mom's letter, that bit of news from the doctor, that time that I wasn't able to do that particular thing for myself. Typically, stressors represent a threat to something we value. It is really the threat with which we cope, not the event. To return to our example of Uncle Ralph, his remark may have threatened your self-esteem, your image of yourself as successful and productive. On the other hand, it may have represented a threat to your relationship with him. Your coping response will be quite different depending upon with which threat you are coping. In the second column of the worksheet, look past the event to what has been threatened. If you are dealing with a couples' issue, your perceptions of the threat may be different, leading you to choose different coping strategies. Identifying your perceptions of the threat may help you to reach a better understanding of each others' feelings and behavior.

The last two columns of the worksheet address coping strategies. First, determine how you formerly coped with similar situations. Usually, this strategy will be unavailable or unworkable now. Once you identify it, however, you may discover that it is still available after all, but perhaps in a somewhat altered form. If not, in the final column, list as many new alternatives as you can, both satisfying and unsatisfying. Listing many alternatives will get your creativity going. Again, the coping alternatives should be chosen to meet the threat in Column Two. Order your alternatives in terms of their desirability. Finally, you may try out some of the coping strategies you list. Talking with Uncle Ralph may not work if his response is a closed one. You may have to move to the second alternative, limiting your contacts with him, in order to preserve your relationship. Employing new coping strategies may take some practice and some support. Let your partner and friends in on your goals, and enlist their support.

There is a final element to stress that requires some attention, as it may block effective problem-solving. Stress may produce anxiety, a form of mismanaged stress that can be momentarily disabling of both rational thought and contact with underlying feelings. As with stress, some anxiety can be a stimulus to action, but in excess it can be immobilizing or interfering. During premature labor, anxiety (usually seen as the result of a stressor) can itself become a stressor. You may worry about anxiety leading to contractions; that is, you may become anxious about being anxious.

Indeed, there are physiological similarities between stress and anxiety responses: increased heart rate, shallowness of breathing, hyperalertness, sleeplessness. It is important to remember that the medications used to control uterine contractions can also produce some of these side effects. Labeling the physiological cues accurately may help reduce secondary anxiety (i.e., worry about being anxious). Dealing with stressful situations directly will also help to ease anxiety. When anxiety interferes with coping, one can invoke relaxation as a means of calming the physiological arousal, making way for clearer insight. Relaxation addresses directly the inhibiting effects of mismanaged stress.

We will close this chapter with a relaxation exercise. While relaxation is particularly useful when stress is experienced acutely in an interfering way, it can become a beneficial aspect of your daily routine as well. For a woman experiencing premature labor it may provide a means of feeling instrumental in efforts to calm her uterus. For her partner it may be a means of achieving a precious few minutes of uncluttered time. If practiced, relaxation can become a finely tuned skill. You can become aware of unneeded tension in your body and learn to relax differential muscle groups unnecessary to the task with which you are involved. In so doing, you expend less wasted energy, reserving it for the activity at hand. This is true with emotional energy as well; emotional tension not channeled through the body is available to deal with emotional stress.

RELAXATION EXERCISE[5]

Choose a quiet place and time, uninterrupted by family needs, telephones, or doorbells. Allow fifteen to thirty minutes for your first session; more or less time may be spent once you know what to do. Lie or sit comfortably. Uncross your arms, legs, and feet. It is best to support your head. Allow your eyes to close. Inhale deeply through your nose. Hold your breath momentarily and then exhale through your mouth, emptying your lungs completely. Repeat this two more times. Focus your attention upon your toes and feet. Tense your toes and feet and hold for a few seconds. Release

---

[5] Adapted from Jacobson, Edmund. *Progressive Relaxation*. Chicago: The University of Chicago Press, 1929.

slowly, feeling each muscle relax. Remember to keep breathing slowly and evenly. Relax the toes and feet fully. Relax more. Feel the difference between the tension and relaxation. Tense your calf and knee. Hold for a few seconds. Slowly release again, feeling the relaxation spread through your knee and calf and through your feet and toes. Continue to tense and flex through the following muscle groups:

— thigh

— buttocks

— abdomen (if you're a pregnant woman, relax only, without tensing)

— chest and shoulders

— arms

— hands and wrists

— neck

— jaw

— face and forehead

After each new muscle group, feel the relaxation spread through all the groups that you have so far tensed and relaxed. At the end, feel the relaxation spread through your entire body. Relax more and more deeply. Enjoy the feeling for as long as you care to before opening your eyes.

Variations:

1. Tense each muscle group twice, focusing your attention on the difference between tension and relaxation.

2. Become aware of how tension in one body part may radiate to other body parts. Get to know how and where your body holds tension, what your patterns are.

3. Concentrate on specific muscle groups that you identify as your critical ones.

4. Alternate tension and relaxation; i.e., relax one arm or leg or an entire side of the body while tensing the other. This helps to create finer control of the relaxation response. For a special challenge, tense your right leg and left arm while relaxing your left leg and right arm, and vice versa.

5. Practice your awareness of tension while involved in your daily activities. Employ muscle tension only where needed to accomplish your task. Relax other muscle groups.

6. Once you are skilled at recognizing tension versus relaxation in your body, you may want to omit the tensing action and concentrate on feeling only the relaxation. Feel it spread from your toes up through your body. (This type of progressive relaxation often seems to promote deeper relaxation in the long run.)

WORKSHEET FOR COPING WITH STRESSORS

Expectant Mother

Event or Stressor	Threat	Old Coping	New Coping Alternatives

WORKSHEET FOR COPING WITH STRESSORS

Partner

Event or Stressor	Threat	Old Coping	New Coping Alternatives

WORKSHEET FOR COPING WITH STRESSORS

Couple

Event or Stressor	Threat	Old Coping	New Coping Alternatives

3

RELATIONSHIPS

The previous chapter addressed issues that challenge a couple sharing a pregnancy with premature labor. Relationships with others as well are affected by, and affect, the premature labor experience. In this chapter, we turn to other intimate relationships with the goal of maximizing understanding and support. We shall discuss relationships with adult family members, most significantly parents. A section on relationships with other children addresses concerns about explaining the situation to small children, dealing with their feelings, and finding alternative ways to spend time with them. A final section on building support networks addresses heretofore undiscussed issues regarding friends, associates, and obstetric personnel. It includes a special note for single parents. Chapter Four is addressed *to* family members in an effort to respond to concerns and feelings they might have.

During your premature labor experience, you may be surprised to discover just how many supportive, caring people you have in your lives. Stressful times can provide an opportunity to become closer; they may also push people apart. Problems will probably arise. You have to decide which relationships are important enough to invest energy toward working out problems. We hope that this chapter can be of help with those relationships in which you choose to put energy.

RELATIONSHIPS WITH
ADULT FAMILY MEMBERS

It seems that about 20 percent of couples in which the woman is confined to bed during premature labor have an adult family member (usually a parent) come to live with them. Others may have family close by, with whom they become more closely involved. Still others may have a family member come for a visit sometime during this period. Adult family members are a major source of help and support for many couples. You may or may not previously have been close to your family or your partner's family. You are, however, likely to be involved in some way now (even if only via your feelings about their lack of involvement). Families are both a wonderful resource and another complicating emotional element in the premature labor experience. Relating in a way that satisfies your mutual needs right now may come relatively easily, or it may take some effort.

Where family is involved, there is the potential for many of the issues discussed in the previous chapters to be encountered by and with them as well. Family members will have their own worries about the baby, feelings of powerlessness and anger. In other words, much of what you may be feeling, they may feel as well. However, their feelings may take a somewhat different form or may not be as well-articulated as yours. Unless they are present on a daily basis, your family will not experience your stresses as centrally as you do, and at times they will not understand. They will use denial more effectively when not in your company, and so perhaps will not even be aware of their fears or feelings. Consequently, you may experience only the indirect manifestations or by-products of their feelings. They may try to maintain their denial, presenting a cheery, chin-up disposition and seeming to ignore your woes. On the other hand, they may be full of advice as a way of dealing with their own feelings of impotence.

So you have one or many third parties emotionally involved at a time of great stress for you. While understanding them and their needs may help you to cope, you probably feel as if you have enough to deal with keeping things together for yourself and your mate. You are bound to feel intensely positive and negative feelings toward your family. At times you may act on these feelings, for better or worse. Old issues in your relationship may reemerge. You may find it comfortable to ease back into being taken care of, or you may feel, intensely, the same disappointments you had as a child. As we suggested in the last chapter, times of stress provide both a danger and an opportunity. While you will inevitably need to use close relationships such as those with your family to vent your feelings, you probably also would like to seize the chance to grow closer. Understanding some of the common elements in this particularly intimate situation may help.

Especially if this is your first child, one factor that cannot be ignored is that of the role transitions being made by yourselves and your parents. You are becoming parents yourselves, striving (if, perhaps, with some ambivalence) to give up some of the child role. Even if you are "mature" expectant parents leading successful adult lives, you will experience some elements of this transition. You may find yourself reexamining and turning away from some of your parents' childrearing styles in favor of your own developing preferences. As a result, you may be especially sensitive when they act in those particularly parental ways toward you. They too must grapple with giving you up as a child—which they may do either reluctantly or with overkill, reacting to their difficulty in doing so. That is, they may be especially parental (in their own style) or they may withdraw from the parent role, insisting that you make your own choices.

The premature labor situation enhances the ambivalences of this normal period of passing the torch. You have been thrust into a somewhat dependent (childlike, if you will) position. As a result, psychological forces are afoot that may render your old parent-child roles more or less attractive for either you or your parents or both. You may particularly want your parents' caretaking at this time, or you may resent needing it. They may feel a familiar tug to protect you, or they may resist the tug in an effort not to intrude. It is a time when your rules for relating are probably undergoing some change and are, therefore, up for grabs. In such a situation, people typically (1) fall back on the old rules, (2) avoid the situation because it is unclear, or (3) gradually create new rules.

If you've had a good relationship with your family, you may ease back into a comfortable give and take. You may find it possible to depend on your parents again in a way that is compatible with their needs as well as yours. You may find a way to tell them what you need differently now.

If there have been some difficulties in your relationship with your family, you may have to work harder to create new rules that are better than the old ones. When a child is in trouble, a parent typically feels responsibility to protect, to "make it better." Their wish to make it better will manifest itself in their usual style, whatever that is. They may be protective; they may take over; they may withdraw, not wanting to be a burden to you or being too afraid of their own feelings. You may have some feelings about their usual style that make it hard to take, especially now. At some point, this may lead to confrontation.

One way to weather such a confrontation is to share with them what you sense about their style of giving, as well as some honest feedback on how they can really be helpful. They too want to be effective in a highly frustrating situation. Only you can tell them what is and isn't helpful.

At some point, you may have to reckon with the fact that your family cannot do what would be helpful—either because they are incapable, or because your expectations were unrealistic. This is a difficult and painful realization. We all like to think that someday our partners and families will provide what we imagine they could, once we or they get it right. Like ourselves, parents have their own fallibilities, and at times are simply unable to meet our expectations of how they "should be." Dealing with your own disappointment now may prepare you for your child's inevitable disappointment in you and free you, in part, from the pressure to be perfect.

Some people, too, feel a sense of failure vis à vis their family at this time. Especially for those pregnant with their first child, this impending birth may give your parents great and obvious joy. You don't want them to be disappointed. In your own right you want to be an independent parent to their beautiful grandchild. Regret over needing them and possibly disappointing them may loom in the back of your mind. Probably this is in part a sincere wish to see them happy, and in part a vestige of an ever-present desire to please your parents. Pleasing your parents may be yet another aspect of the fantasized pregnancy that has been lost to you. You may, however, gain something by dealing with reality. Instead of acting on assumptions of the past about what is necessary to make you or your parents happy, you have the opportunity and the challenge to get down to basics and really examine what is important to yourselves and each other.

A specific issue that sometimes arises for couples in premature labor is what to do about the family member who doubts or disagrees with obstetric opinion. In their wish to be supportive, family members may overidentify, recalling the conditions of their own pregnancies in an effort to assume that theirs were the same as yours are now. Such a family member may either minimize or magnify the risks of your premature labor. They may insist that you don't need to be in bed. They may urge you to seek a second opinion, often from their "approved" expert. It may be helpful to remind them and yourselves that the improved success of obstetrics in preventing premature birth is quite recent. Indeed, in previous years, premature labor was rarely detected, and for this reason fewer women were confined to bed. Indeed, too, many more babies were born prematurely with dire results. Such well-meaning but unhelpful family members can confuse the medical picture by bringing indirect pressure to bear or sabotaging direct communication. Your practitioner will deal best with you directly. Decide how *you* feel about your treatment, and then gently insist to the family member that you feel confident about how it is being handled. Share with them excerpts from this book. Suggest that their support in helping you to carry out what you need to do would be appreciated, but that at the very least their doubts should be curtailed, because they undermine your ability to proceed as you deem appropriate.

Finally, where families are concerned, there are, of course, in-laws. Your partner may have an idea of how the foregoing discussion pertains to her or his parents; but to you, your in-laws (and dealing with them) may be a relative mystery, since you know them less well. If it is your in-law that has come to live or visit, you may receive a crash course in family dynamics complete with *in vivo* experience. Absorbing a little-known family member into your usually private daily routines and activities, and what's more, asking that they pitch in, can feel awkward. Your partner (whose parent it is) should do most of the interfacing where possible until you get comfortable. You will have to forge your own brand of relationship and perhaps deal with some of the issues discussed above.

In deciding which family member might come to help out (if you have a choice), consider what it is you need right now and who might best fit in. The ideal live-in family member might be someone who

— is comfortable taking over responsibilities

— respects your style and wishes

— is self-entertaining

— understands your need for private time, both individually and as a couple

— is optimistic and emotionally accessible

— supports wholeheartedly the relationship between you and your partner.

Most relatives will not be so ideal. Consider which aspects are most important to you right now.

At some point during your experience, you may encounter conflicts with your partner over relations with in-laws. It is a time when you both need nurturance, and you may disagree over how your families provide it. You both want to feel close to your families right now, and thus may be protective and a little defensive about them. Or you may find yourself preferring your in-laws' styles and feeling guilty or disappointed in regard to your own family. It may help to see your families' styles of giving not as "better" or "worse," but as different. Certainly it is a time when you can afford to rate highly your own needs and take advantage of the giving that meets them right now. At the same time, you undoubtedly will want to preserve and build good feelings among all your family members so as not to strain future relationships. In fact, if you are able to take advantage now of this opportunity to develop and stabilize significant family relationships, the investment will be invaluable in the years to come once the baby is born and begins to flourish within a comfortable extended family structure.

We hope that the comments offered here will help you to develop your family relationships in positive directions. We encourage you to use the following chapter, "For the Family," as a means of opening communication and promoting understanding with your family at this time. Please share the information contained therein with those who want or need to know more.

RELATIONSHIPS
WITH YOUR CHILDREN

> *"I feel as if you are dead, Mom, since you have been in the hospital away from me now for two weeks. The only positive thing is that when I come to visit you, suddenly you come alive for me for a little while."*
>
> Lukas Haas, (eight years), whose
> mother was hospitalized for
> three weeks in premature labor with twins.

If you already have children at home, you are no doubt frequently torn between the needs of those already born and those yet to be born. As we noted earlier, this conflict is likely to heighten your ambivalence and make compliance with bedrest requirements seem more difficult. In this section, we shall address three aspects of relating to children in the family with premature labor: (1) explaining why Mommy has to lie down, (2) understanding the child's changeable behavior and feelings, and (3) staying involved in the child's daily activities.

For the couple with other children, additional help in the form of daycare, babysitters, friends, or family becomes essential. This may entail an additional change in routine for your child. In choosing what form of additional help to use, you will have to weigh several factors, including finances, your amount of living space, and the needs of your child. Of course, for your child's sake, it is ideal to minimize the number of changes as much as possible. It would be difficult for the home-reared preschooler to begin daycare at this time, although a transition to half-day preschool might be feasible if a familiar adult could also attend for awhile. An older child, better able to verbalize about the circumstances, might handle an addition of after-school daycare. The option most frequently chosen is having an adult family member come to live with you for awhile.

Regardless of how you choose to meet your child's needs for supervision and physical caretaking, you will want to maximize your child's understanding of the situation. Of course, how you explain Mommy's need to be in bed right now will depend on the age of your child and what works best for you. Here we provide only a few general guidelines:

Don't tell your child that Mommy is sick. Mommy has already been lost to some extent, and further loss may be feared. Children frequently associate illness with discomfort, and therefore may worry about Mommy's well-being. Be attentive to signs of clingingness as possible indicators of fears of losing Mommy. Offer reassurance that Mommy is and will be fine and that your child will not be sent away.

Do offer an age-appropriate version of the truth. Your child probably knows by now that a brother or sister is on the way. If not, now is the time for explanations. The Bibliography lists some excellent illustrated books for helping children to understand birth and their feelings about it. Explain in some way that Mommy has to stay in bed so that the baby won't be born too soon—before it is big enough. Later additional explanations might address the following facts:

1. This is a special problem (not every Mommy has to stay in bed with another baby).

2. There was a problem with Mommy's body not holding the baby in tightly enough. Perhaps you could illustrate with a drawing or use a sock with a hole in the toe and insert something heavy enough to slide through, including some "contractions" (or "squeezes") to help it do so. Illustrate that it will not fall through when the sock is horizontal and when there are no "squeezes." You will no doubt need to follow through to assure your child that the baby wouldn't just fall out quickly. In other words, Mommy's trips to the bathroom are OK, but in general, she needs to lie down to keep her uterus from "squeezing."

Tell your child a little at a time. Enough should be said to satisfy your child's curiosity but not be overwhelming. Repeat yourself often. As you no doubt know, a child's mind can interpret your crystal-clear explanations in the oddest ways. You will be most successful if your explanations are short and in response to questions. Your child will let you know when more information is needed. You may need to be alert for signs of misunderstanding, however, such as concern about your trips to the bathroom.

Assure your child that it is no one's fault. The impending birth of a sibling is an event full of ambivalences. While most children will at times be excited about the prospect, it is a safe bet that they also sometimes wish to get rid of the encroacher. Preschool children especially tend to think magically and egocentrically. Your child may think that "hateful" thoughts toward the fetus have caused this situation, and feel guilty as a result. If your child is being especially helpful and concerned, or especially withdrawn, you might consider this as a possibility. Your explanation that there was a problem with Mommy's body will help, but so will your direct assurances. The need for repeated hospitalization or other mini-setbacks may similarly stir up a child's feelings of responsibility; be sensitive to this as a possibility.

Employ your child's imagination. Children of all ages love stories and they learn much from them. A child will be better able to identify with the fetus when told stories about your pregnancy with him or her. Together with your child imagine the baby. Give the baby characteristics that your child can understand. Talk together to the baby as a way of encouraging the baby to stay inside the womb.

KATHLEEN'S STORY FOR
HER DAUGHTER, MIRANDA

I am currently on full-time bedrest, taking Terbutaline for premature labor at sixteen weeks of gestation. My daughter, Miranda, is three and a half years old. I was also on bedrest with her, along with medication, and delivered her at term. I explain to Miranda, with the following story, why I am lying down all day. She likes me to tell her the story at least ten times a day: she often pats my stomach or places her head on it when I tell the story.

Once upon a time, there was a tiny tiny baby in Mommy's tummy. This baby was in a hurry to be born before it was time to be born. So Mommy went to the doctor who knows about babies before they are born and said: "Doctor, my tiny baby is impatient and doesn't want to wait its turn to be born: what should I do?"

The doctor said: "Go home and rest in bed and maybe you can teach the baby to be patient so the baby can wait until its turn to be born." So

Mommy went home and rested and rested. Every day she put her hands on her tummy and said: "Little baby, please be patient and wait your turn to be born."

And so the baby waited and was born in the hospital at the right time. Now that little baby was you.

Now it's time for Mommy and Daddy to have another baby. This baby is impatient, just like you were. So Mommy's doctor said that I have to go home and rest and rest and teach the tiny baby to be patient. And so that is why Mommy has to stay in bed now. Help me teach the baby to be patient and wait its turn. Can you talk to the baby and ask the baby to be patient?

Kathleen Bartle, mother
of Miranda, age three years

Just as you will, your child will experience the gamut of emotions. In some ways, a child's feelings may be more obvious; in some ways, less. But you can expect your youngster to be concerned and to wish to help, and your explanations will ease the worry. Allowing children to help in some tangible ways will also help them to deal with their own feelings of powerlessness. Your child may initiate ways of helping, or you might suggest some. Certainly children can bring things to Mommy, carry messages to other family members, help Daddy with chores, even stroke Mommy's tummy or talk to the baby. Your child might enjoy having a blank book, to draw pictures of the baby as the baby grows.

Periods of helpfulness may alternate with periods of disengagement from Mommy. Your child may merely seem to ignore you, quickly forming an attachment to an alternate caretaker, or may more actively resist your efforts to relate. Your child is struggling with the difficult task of giving up a great deal of your availability and active companionship, a necessity over which there is no control. One way a child can gain control is to become the one who is giving *you* up. This may be difficult to take at a time when you already feel sad about not being able to do the many things with and for your child that you would like. A comment about your own sadness may help, but in general you will probably have to tolerate some periods of withdrawal, making the effort to remain open should your child choose to respond.

Anger at parents and at the fetus may take a number of forms. "Daddy doesn't do it like Mommy does." "Why can't you get up just this once, Mommy." "I don't want a brother anyway." Your child didn't want the familiar world disrupted, and will probably let you know that the change is not satisfactory. At times the expression of these feelings may be aggressive, probably more often verbally than physically. Although physical aggression toward people or property cannot be allowed, there are ways for it to be expressed appropriately. You may want to channel it into such activities as doll play or drawing. Children express themselves well to and through imaginary characters—even Mr. Thumbkin, if no one else is handy. Talking to an understanding imaginary figure who also has feelings, or who can tell a story about a child who did, helps children to identify with someone on their own level.

Finally, your child may go through periods of regression, when behavior long since outgrown reappears. The toilet-trained child may wet again. The cup drinker may want a bottle. The sound sleeper may wake in the night. The sophisticated talker may adopt an earlier, babyish style of speech. Or your child may simply resist forward movement, not wanting to take on anything new. By unconsciously regressing in these ways, children try to assure themselves that their needs to depend on you will be met, that they are still their parents' children and will be cared for as such. Generally, a tolerant attitude to such regressions, with perhaps an occasional (but not overdone) comment about how good it feels to be taken care of, will help them to get the needed reassurance. In time, your child will be ready to move forward again developmentally.

Although having split allegiances will be hard for you as parents, children generally do profit from witnessing their parents' concern and care for a sibling. Some part of them identifies with the sibling and is reminded that, indeed, they themselves are cared for and valued. You need not hesitate to love your unborn child in your child's presence. Neither do you need to give up all the ways you had of loving your already born child. Here are some suggestions for keeping involved in your child's life despite having to stay in bed or having limited time.

— Try to maintain a family dinner hour, even if it's around the living-room coffee table or in the bedroom. Dinner can be an important way of sharing good feelings and talking about the day's events. It also lends a sense of routine that can be counted on.

— Share your nesting area with your child for special activities: have a supply of storybooks, drawing paper, and games nearby. One mother on bedrest enclosed the living room with child-proof gates so that she and her toddler son could share the entire living room as their nest together at certain times during the day.

— If Mom has to be hospitalized, check on visitation policy. If a visit is not possible, a picture of Mommy at the hospital can assuage a child's fearful fantasies. There may be little things that can be sent home (e.g., bedside accessories) to help a child feel involved. Likewise, your child may want to send things to Mommy.

— When the child is out with another caretaker, have pictures taken of the activities to bring home to Mommy and/or Daddy. A camera that develops film immediately is ideal for this. Drawing pictures can be another way of sharing the day. Pictures give the young child who lacks verbal and abstract skills a concrete way to share their lives.

MOTHERING AARON
WHILE ON BEDREST

One week after my son's second birthday, I was diagnosed as being in premature labor. I was twenty-two weeks pregnant. For the next month, we experimented with varying levels of activity and watched my cervix continue to efface. Finally at twenty-six weeks I was put down for complete bedrest for the rest of the pregnancy.

The most painful aspect of the premature labor experience for me was losing the ability to be my son's main caretaker at such a critical time in his development. I felt as though all my careful work could be washed away, and that he would feel both abandoned by me and assaulted by an insensitive and haphazard world.

Even after I had set up what was as close to an ideal situation as possible—Aaron's grandmother, a neighborhood teenager, and my husband all filled in—I found myself suffering. I missed watching Aaron grow. And although everyone was very respectful of my instructions and comments about Aaron's existence, I knew there was a gaping hole in his life too. I began to notice subtle changes in his behavior that were hard to interpret—so much was happening to him that I didn't know whether he was simply responding as any two-year-old would, or was reacting to my bedrest, or was frustrated about something that had just happened.

The two changes that concerned me the most were intense mood shifts accompanied by dramatic gestures, and a tendency to clam up, get a funny look on his face, and run out of the room when something bothered him.

I discovered that there was usually one of three emotional states underlying any of his unusual behaviors:

anger: usually at my inability to get up and provide for him;

fear: of losing me, or that my condition was permanent;

rejection: by me; that bedrest meant I didn't want to be with him.

His angry feelings usually manifested themselves in the exaggerated gestures, while his fearful and rejected feelings made him silent and solitary. What I wanted most was for him to be able to express his feelings and get whatever reassurance and comfort he needed.

Several things helped us dissipate the tensions of this time and kept our communication fluent, as well as giving us the intimate time we were both missing.

We had direct conversations about what was happening to me—conversations in which I told him I would get better and be able to do everything with him again; that I loved him and wanted to be able to play with him, and fix his food, and give him baths, etc. These conversations all helped, but only to a certain degree. Conversations only go so far, and are easily forgotten by an active two-year-old. What he really needed was time spent with me on activities both fun and healing.

1. *Books, books, books.* Aaron tended to gravitate toward books that dealt indirectly and gently with his concerns, such as loss of mother *(Are You My Mother?* by Dr. Seuss) and confinement to bed *(1, 2, 3 with Ant and Bee,* by Angela Banner). The latter is a book in which Ant is put to bed and gets MAD about having to stay there. On that particular page, we put the book down and pounded the bed with our fists and yelled about how mad we were about our current situation. Aaron LOVED this: I think seeing me get mad validated his feelings and made it OK for him to express himself. I imagine children of all ages can find books, or be helped to find books, which are helpful in this way.

2. *Blocks, Legos, Tinker Toys.* Creating environments and objects on the bed is especially helpful when miniature figures are incorporated: men, women, dogs, cats. Aaron revealed lots of his feelings about our situation through play with the Lego people. He also made a lot of beds with his blocks.

3. *Aggression games.* We used toys like cash registers, typewriters, hammer/nail kits—things the child can pound and hit unself-consciously, just to release some of the physical side of the anger. Obviously, more aggression games can take place with other family members, off the bed and out of doors.

4. *Balloon kick and blow.* Aaron is very active and it seemed important to find some active games I could participate in with him. Besides, I love the squeals and laughter of this kind of play. *The Balloon Kick:* The child lies on their back between parents on the bed. The parents bat the balloon in the air space above the child's feet. Child kicks gleefully at the balloon. The parents, especially the partner, keep the balloon within the boundaries of the bed. *The Balloon Blow:* The parent blows up the balloon and hands it to the child untied. The child releases the balloon and chases it all over the room.

5. *Pretending.* Aaron pretended to be many things on the bed—an Olympic swimmer (he takes his marks and dives onto the bed, swims a length, and is "the winner"), a gymnast (tricks on the bed), a baby (lots of hugs and lullabies), a dog, etc. All children have their own "pretends," but I wrote this down because it was one of the ways I could be inside a world with Aaron, sharing and creating as we went. Sometimes we took trips together, and the things he invented (like me being the baby, him taking me to the doctor, him being the doctor) really informed me of his inner workings.

6. *Drawing, cutting, gluing.* Arts and crafts can be done in bed. I kept a big paper bag full of paper, glue, scissors, stamps, scraps of cloth, old calendar pages, sequins, ribbon, macaroni, and dried beans by the bed. Sometimes I'd hang our finished creations on the door. We did this several times a day. We also changed the sheets more frequently than we used to!

We ended up spending about two to three hours (in one- to one-and-a-half-hour increments) alone together each day. This seemed to satisfy the hunger in me for active participation with Aaron, and kept his emotions more even. And there were benefits to this forced weaning: Aaron became much closer to both his grandmother and his father, which has sustained him through the early days of his sister's arrival; I've learned to be less controlling and hovering in relation to him; and I've seen strength of character and flexibility develop in all of us by the demands of this time.

Laura Landon, mother of Aaron (two years)
and Emily (three months).

BUILDING AND USING
SUPPORT NETWORKS

Among your circle of associations—family, friends, religious and work associates, neighbors, obstetric practitioners—you may be surprised at who lends support and who does not. Often help can come from the least expected source, while on the other hand you may be disappointed that those you expected to be involved are not. Who will fall into which category defies prediction. The response of others will depend upon a complex combination of their own past experiences, their feelings about your situation, their availability, and your messages to them. It is this latter area which we will address.

What can be said, really, is very brief. Appreciate and respect your own needs for help and for autonomy. Let others know how they can fit in. You may be a phone talker or a people person. (One mother confined to bed scheduled friends for lunch every day for weeks in advance.) On the other hand, you may prefer time alone and only reluctantly rely on others at this time. For you, making calls will be more of an effort. It may help to let people know this, and to be very welcoming when their calls come in.

Couples in premature labor may find it helpful to be in touch with other couples who are either currently in the same situation or have experienced it in the past. One or the other of these options may be more attractive to you. Someone who has similar experience will likely be as involved as you are in medication dosages, weeks gestation, managing your physical space, etc. You are consumed with these details; someone with first-hand experience will be too, and will want to talk about them as much as you do. Still, sharing a similar experience may be the only way in which you are alike; the person whose name you are given to call may not be a good match for you in either style or experience. You may want different things from your contacts. If you are disappointed in your first effort, don't hesitate to ask your practitioner for another name, explaining what it is you're looking for. You didn't choose your friends out of the phone book, and finding a simpatico phone buddy is also not a casual accomplishment.

Putting you in touch with other couples and other resources is one way in which you can ask your practitioner for help. We encourage you to be assertive in getting your needs met in other ways as well. Certainly you have a right to medical information, including alternatives for treatment and what the future may hold. In all likelihood, you will work out a mutually respectful relationship with your practitioner. At times, though, you may find yourself angry at and resistant to your practitioner, or alternatively, submissive and eager to please. Some reflection on the situation, perhaps with your partner, may help you to understand the source of these attitudes. In this culture medical practitioners are seen as experts. As such, they can sometimes slip into an authoritative stance that may seem to exclude the patient. On the other hand, patients frequently bring to the relationship with their doctor all their usual feelings about authority. When your communication with your practitioner is blocked to the point where your treatment is threatened, it is time to sort out the source of the trouble.

Finally, a few words for one for whom the premature labor experience is especially difficult—the single mother. Having a baby without a partner has inherent lonely moments and stresses. You certainly didn't bargain for this. If earlier you had questioned the wisdom of your decision, now you may feel that this is an outright sign that you made a mistake, or that it is nature's way of toughening you up to face single parenthood. Of course, these conclusions are no more true for you than for the partnered parent.

Not having a primary partner, you will be especially reliant upon your support network, and you may have to deal with some particular sensitivities. Certain of your associates may have disapproved of your decision to have this baby. They may now be out-and-out righteous about it, or seem quietly judgmental; just what you don't need.

Many single parents report pressures (both internal and external) to be a "super-parent." You have to "do it all," "handle it all"—more so than the partnered parent. You may experience premature labor in that light: "I chose this, so I'm not going to complain." By feeling that you have to be tough, you will cut off the range of emotions you can be expected, and indeed need, to have, just as does the partnered woman.

For the single parent, premature labor may be less a matter of being tough than of choosing your supports particularly well and turning away from unhelpful or even hurtful ones. Hopefully, you will find one or two trustworthy confidantes, and will make contact with other women in premature labor. The present time might be an excellent opportunity to explore the resources in your community that offer special support to a woman choosing single parenthood (e.g., contact the local women's center to find out about support groups, etc.).

4

FOR THE FAMILY:
RELATING TO THE COUPLE
IN PREMATURE LABOR

Whether at a distance or nearby, the family members of a couple experiencing premature labor frequently have questions and concerns about the situation that may not get addressed. Indeed, until recently, medical personnel were the only source to whom couples themselves could turn for supportive information. This book is written in an attempt to remedy that. Our goal is to bring to couples and their families information about the medical and psychosocial factors involved in premature labor. We believe it to be a highly stressful time for all concerned. By sharing with you common medical knowledge as well as supportive information based on the insights of other families, we hope to promote optimism and a more comfortable experience for everyone concerned.

We are aware from observation and personal experience that the families of premature labor patients frequently play a critical role in the treatment. That is, they can have both a tangible and an intangible influence on the ease of confinement to bed, keeping the household in working order, and staying sane. We often feel as if a vital part of the forces affecting the pregnancy is at home, while we sit in the office. This section is written in recognition of your role at this time and of the questions and concerns you might have as well. While we won't summarize here the medical and practical information given in other chapters, we do encourage you to read as much of this entire book as you wish. Here we will discuss some of the issues that tend to arise for couples in premature labor and their families. Our intent is to clarify for you what the common stressors of premature labor are, how couples may deal with them emotionally, and how you might help. We also hope to speak to some of the feelings family members typically have in relation to the situation.

First, what is premature labor? Premature labor is diagnosed when a woman experiences regular, measurable contractions that produce changes in the cervix. If labor progresses, there is the threat that the baby will be born before maturity, with significant risk to health and survival. In recent years, great advances have been made in detecting preterm labor and preventing premature birth. Approximately 6 to 8 percent of all pregnant women develop premature labor. Treatment includes varying amounts of bedrest, and sometimes medication to calm the uterine contractions. Some women who have had problems with cervical change earlier in their pregnancy may be given a cerclage (stitch) to close the cervical opening. Hospitalization is sometimes required to monitor and gain control of contractions, but usually, a woman may remain at home, with regular medical visits and educated self-monitoring. Chapter One of this book provides more extensive medical information regarding premature labor and incompetent cervix.

The fear of early delivery, together with restriction of activity and its consequences, poses many stressors for the pregnant couple and for family members. Chapter Two details these stressors as they are commonly experienced by the couple. We shall briefly summarize them here, along with some commentary about the parallel experiences that family members frequently have.

Worries about the baby come and go for all concerned, and may be expressed directly and indirectly. The latter may include preoccupation with the woman's body (contractions, fetal movement, weight gain), information-seeking, and even ambivalence toward the baby. Periods of worry and tears may alternate with periods of denial, in which potential dangers are seemingly ignored. Some of this is to be expected, and indeed is frequently helpful in coping with worry. Denial can at times, however, result from inability to face one's fears about premature birth. At some point, most couples (and perhaps family members) find it relieving to confront their fears and get some information about the consequences of premature birth. Chapter Seven and the Bibliography at the end of this book suggest some sources for doing so.

Denial is not the same as suppression of worry. Many family members seem to feel that they don't want to heighten the couple's worry or "hold a bad thought," and so attempt to limit their own concerns and questions. You certainly have your own hopes for the healthy birth of a new family member in addition to your desire for the couple to be happy. You are bound to worry. Most couples report that they appreciate some honest discussion of worries with their loved ones. By discussing them, you come to know what is in one another's minds and to deal with reality, rather than relegating concerns to speculation and fearful fantasies. Timing is, of course, an issue in such discussions. A family member who is upset usually profits from serious consideration, exploration, and sharing of their concerns, along with some encouragement. A family member in a period of denial may slough off discussion of worries and not be open to sharing.

The loss of career and/or household roles for the woman and increased duties for her partner challenge a couple's usual way of relating, threatening to throw them into emotional and organizational disarray. Indeed, you may arrive on the scene at just such a time, and fear the worst. Rest assured that with patience from all a new equilibrium will be found. There may be an initial or midway period when one or both of the couple just want to be taken care of. For the most part, though, it is important for the confined pregnant woman to discover ways in which she can still do the things that matter most to her. She may still need to feel herself in control of her household, effective as a parent, valued as a confidante. In this regard, it is important for her family members not to take over too much. Knowing what is too much or too little is in part an intuitive endeavor, fueled by your sensitive knowledge of your loved ones' needs. On the other hand, it is not done by magic. The right balance will emerge slowly, and may even change over time. Without a doubt, striking that balance will from time to time require frank discussion.

Both the woman in premature labor and her partner have to struggle with feelings of dependency and powerlessness. Needing others to help out is frequently hard for them to accept. Finding ways to regain control over daily routines, self-care, and the health of the baby becomes very important. At some point in the premature labor experience, women especially tend to experience depression as a result of feeling helpless and unproductive. Partners too may begin to feel inadequate to the tasks required, especially if their overload leads to lowered job or personal performance. For everyone, including family, there may be a recurring sense of helplessness, especially during times when it is difficult to get the contractions under control.

As a family member, your position is uniquely sensitive. You want so much to be helpful—and indeed there are many ways in which you can be. Ultimately, however, it is not your pregnant body and not your household. From the "outside" you may see things that you would handle quite differently, but know that it is not within your power or purview to do so. You walk the fine line between being helpful and respectful—not always an easy line to discern. It may be especially difficult to discern now, due in part to the emotions surrounding the birth of a child—especially a first child. If the couple is having their first child and you are a parent of one of the couple, you are all dealing with a change in life positions. Your child is becoming a parent, and is growing less childlike. This period of passing the torch is full of ambivalences. It is wonderful to anticipate sharing yet another realm of adulthood with your adult child, and yet sad to give up another bit of the past. For your child, it may be both attractive and painful to become still more responsible and independent. The dependency that premature labor entails adds yet another complication. You may find your child wishing to recapture for one last luxurious time the experience of being cared for by you before becoming the caretaker. On the other hand, your child's struggle to define personal attitudes as a prospective parent may lead to seemingly irrational rejections of your efforts to provide help. Just acknowledging that this transition is occurring and is an emotional factor may help in dealing with family feelings at this time.

If you live at a distance from the couple, you may feel especially helpless or frustrated in your efforts to understand and provide support. Just as we recommend that the couple arm themselves with as much information as possible to combat their feelings of powerlessness, we suggest a similar route for family members. Information about the medical prospects and alternatives helps everyone to feel more in control. Likewise, frequent contact with the couple about their progress and needs may help you to discern better just how you can be helpful.

Anger is an expected and important emotion for all concerned. There is much about the situation that is difficult to accept. Expressing anger indicates that one is involved and still vital, rather than passive and depressed. As there is no easily identifiable target for angry feelings related to premature labor, they may at times become ventilated among family members over seemingly unrelated issues. Everyone is disappointed and to some degree anxious. Everyone would like their loved ones, who *usually* make things all better again, to make things all better this time too, while knowing that they can't. Family members usually have a history of weathering angry disagreements, and so may provide a safe arena for angry outbursts now. Anger directed toward you from the couple may focus on issues of how you involve yourself or try to be helpful. It may have a flavor familiar from past arguments. Frequently, the anger that emerges during stressful periods of change stems from old issues that are now coming to a head. Indeed, such stressful, intense times as these provide an opportunity to clarify and resolve old feelings.

There are two additional stressors that frequently affect the couple in premature labor. Merely knowing that these stressors may form a background to tensions at this time can prove helpful to family members. First, couples in premature labor commonly experience financial strain. Adding to the strain, money concerns may be difficult for a couple to discuss even with each other because they seem either overwhelming or "petty" in relation to concerns for the baby. Yet financial control is vital to feeling secure, especially in a time of insecurity when little indulgences are especially needed. Second, for many couples, sexual activity is restricted, often adding an additional edge of tension to the situation. Clinical attention to a woman's body can make her feel depersonalized and "like an incubator." It is important for couples to find alternative ways of sharing intimacy and affection.

Finally, there is disappointment for all concerned that the pregnancy has not turned out as imagined. Pregnancy is typically a time of great family joy and excitement, including shopping for the baby and decorating a nursery. The couple may have looked forward to particular ways of sharing their last few childless months—perhaps a trip, at least some active moments. If they have other children, they may feel deprived of fun times with them before the new arrival. The couple's "fantasy" pregnancy might also have included images of your pleasure in sharing the experience. They may even worry, consciously or unconsciously, that they have disappointed you, robbing you of some joy and leaving you with fear. In part this may be true. You may have had to change plans, coming to visit earlier than expected for a far less joyful reason. You may have looked forward to sharing the shopping, the preparations, the baby shower. There is loss in this. Yet there are other, if less traditional, ways to share the planning and the joy. Family members can be a great help in scoping out alternatives in baby equipment and clothes. You can send or bring information back to the couple for their decisions—descriptions of strollers, brochures on baby furniture, samples of wallpaper or paint. What a tremendous help to the time-rich woman and her time-impoverished partner!

Although helping out before the birth may not be personally "as much fun" as if the baby were already born, your contribution to the baby's health now is profound. There is no more meaningful gift to give your grandchild or new family member than helping the pregnancy continue to term. To begin life as a healthy newborn after a long, complex pregnancy rather than a premature six- or seven-month baby in the Intensive Care Nursery ensures the greatest potential for the newborn's survival and quality of life.

It is important, we feel, to acknowledge the real disappointments of premature labor as a first step toward inventing new ways of achieving what was imagined for the pregnancy. It is important to remember that, with proper treatment, many women who experience premature labor do deliver healthy, full-term babies. Couples, and perhaps family members as well, sometimes, in normal emotional self-defense, close off their feelings of attachment to the fetus. We encourage them gradually to recapture such feelings. As the pregnancy progresses, we encourage all involved to express and participate in the excitement and joy of preparations for the expected one. The pregnancy is not as it was imagined to be, but it still *is* —with all of its miracles and promise.

Indeed, while there are many stressors in the premature labor experience, there are positive aspects to dwell upon as well. First, of course, there is optimism from the fact that the early labor was detected and is, in all probability, treatable. In addition, many couples report that the premature labor experience was ultimately a personally and interpersonally strengthening time, as crisis times often are. There certainly are increased opportunities to rely upon and become close to family members, to overcome old problems and discover new ways of relating. Both women and their partners sometimes discover or rediscover personal assets that perhaps were previously underused but that emerge under these circumstances. One of the greatest challenges of the situation is, in fact, to find some meaningfulness in it—to glimpse the opportunities involved as well as to acknowledge the stresses and strains.

In closing, we provide a list of ways in which couples have said that family members can be helpful. They may or may not be on your couple's list, but they may give you some ideas for discussion.

How Family Members May Help:

— Be interested. Let them know you are concerned and want to be informed on a regular basis. Such contact provides an outlet for the need to talk about the experiences involved and makes it easier to share details. Try to call frequently and, if geographically possible, make regular visits. The time spent now in developing a closer relationship will be an excellent investment in a continuing one once the new family member has arrived.

— Be concerned. Acknowledge the seriousness of the situation and recognize that the worries are real. By doing so you support the couple's hard work and sacrifices for the welfare of their baby.

— Be optimistic. Don't hesitate to respond to the couple's hopefulness and to anticipate the birth of a healthy baby.

— Be real. Acknowledge your own fears and disappointments, using your own best judgment of when and how it is appropriate to do so. Also using judgment, let the couple know when they get on your nerves.

More concretely, you might do some of the following, depending on your proximity and availability of time.

— Send magazines and used books.

— Send "care packages" of homemade treats or canned goods (please minimize the sugars).

— Collect information about and samples of baby equipment, wallpapers, etc., for the couple to "shop at home."

— Take their shopping list and do the footwork.

— Stock their freezer with home-cooked foods wrapped in serving sizes.

— Remind the couple that they are doing a great job (if they are), and that you are proud of how they are handling the situation (if you are).

— Take the other children on outings so that Mom and Dad can have some quiet time together.

— Take over a regular chore (mowing the lawn, picking up other children from school).

— Share with them whatever your special brand of giving is.

THANKS FOR HELPING YOUR COUPLE TO HOLD ON!

FLORENCE'S STORY:
A GRANDMOTHER'S PERSPECTIVE

It's not easy becoming a grandmother. It was a happy moment when I heard that my daughter Elysa was pregnant with her first child. I was filled with gladness. I remembered my own joy of having three wonderful babies. But with this gladness came an unspoken fear. Many years ago I delivered a dead full-term baby. My fear was for my daughter. Might this happen to her? Will something go wrong to harm her happiness? I tried to rid myself of these thoughts, but they stayed to haunt me for months to come.

Elysa's pregnancy was going well. She was feeling fine and continued her daily business routine. With this good news, my fears began to fade.

When Elysa was in her eighth month, she started to have premature contractions. Her doctor advised complete bedrest, in the hope that she could hold back the birth until full term. Elysa was concerned and alarmed at the thought of an early delivery. While I tried (long distance) to ease her anxieties, my fears returned to torment me. My insides hurt for the want to be with her, to give her the care only I could give. There I was on the opposite coast. I was unable to do more than to call once or twice a day.

The following six to seven weeks were the most emotional, unnerving time of my life. I kept pushing the days along—I could not wait for each day to be over, so that I could push the next day into the past. My daily thoughts were about her physical health and her emotional well-being. I cursed the miles that separated us.

Well, everything does come to an end, and for me it was a happy ending. Elysa held on for eleven days beyond her full-term due date, delivered with a saddleblock anesthetic, and had a healthy, beautiful girl—Jamie. Today Elysa is a happy healthy mother, Jamie is a wonderful child, and I am a most happy grandmother, with a few more of the gray hairs that come with living and loving.

Florence G. Blatt,
grandmother of Jamie, (one year).

5

MAXIMIZING TIME AND SPACE

*by Peggy Henning Berlin, Ph.D.,
and Joan and Lee Zukor[1]*

The preceding chapters have dealt with the many and varied emotional aspects of the premature labor experience. This chapter will deal with the practical aspects—the "how to's" during your confinement to bed. The suggestions presented here come from couples previously in premature labor. Hopefully they will stimulate your own creativity to invent strategies that will make your experience more satisfying.

TIME

Time is an interesting commodity: both absolute and relative, made finite by our schedules and yet infinite by its nature. It is perhaps the only resource equally available to all people. You will both no doubt reflect upon time quite a bit during your experience with premature labor, cursing at times its snail's pace and at times its speed in slipping through your fingers. You want to extend your baby's time in the womb, and yet you probably would like your confinement to be over as soon as possible.

From time immemorial, humankind has made the marking of time a central and even sacred activity. By doing so we remind ourselves both of the finite nature of our lives on this planet and of our place in the continuous, repetitive, and evolving motion of seasons and generations. Marking time helps us to accomplish what we need to survive, whether it be plant-

---

[1] Joan and Lee Zukor are the parents of Adam, age one, who was born at term after fourteen weeks of bedrest.

ing, harvesting, and storing, or more modern versions thereof. Marking time in broader strokes enables us to reflect upon how our present experience fits into the larger scheme of our lives and the lives of others. By marking time we attempt—and indeed in many ways are able—to achieve some control, some predictability, and some perspective over our lives. And yet there is another way to deal with time: by being at once in it and outside it, by being in the present moment. In this section we hope to address these multiple aspects of time as they relate to the premature labor experience—a time when time itself is a most precious commodity.

As was noted in Chapter Two, the woman in premature labor and her partner will have to deal with an obvious dichotomy in their perceptions of time. The expectant mother will probably perceive an excess of time on her hands—time abundance. Her busy partner, on the other hand, will perceive that there is too little time—time pressure. Indeed, time does continue at its own pace, despite our efforts to hurry or slow it. The task, therefore, is not to manage *time,* but to manage *ourselves* with respect to time.

TIME ABUNDANCE

Time abundance is the feeling of wanting time to pass more quickly, usually experienced as a need to "fill" time that is unstructured or unscheduled. It is often experienced when one is waiting for something to pass—such as the weeks until your baby's delivery is considered "safe." The same amount of time is left in your pregnancy as if you were not in premature labor, but now it seems oh so much longer. If you are confined to bed, many of the activities with which you both filled and marked your time are suddenly impossible. Getting up and carrying out your daily routine lent regularity and progression to your life. Without these familiar activities, time can seem to crawl. Both you and your partner probably had goal points scattered through your pregnancy to psychologically mark your progress: at sixteen weeks possibly an amniocentesis, at thirty weeks a childbirth education class, at thirty-five weeks a shower, at some point buying equipment and decorating a nursery. Now you may find it difficult to anticipate these milestones, either because they seem unfeasible under your circumstances, or because your worry about the baby makes you either too superstitious about thinking far ahead or too focused on the more immediate goals of extending the pregnancy. Without some smaller goals, the remaining weeks of your pregnancy may seem to extend forever. We will therefore suggest some practical ways of marking and filling time both within any given day and over the course of the pregnancy.

Establishing New Routines

Each of you will need to restructure your daily routines. To do so will take some experimenting and deciding about priorities. We will discuss strategies for partners in the section to follow about time pressure. Here we will address the pregnant woman's need to create new patterns.

> *I always told myself I'd love a couple of months with nothing to do. Somehow, counting the little balls on my chenille bedspread wasn't exactly what I'd had in mind!*
>
> *Expectant Mother*

The first week of your confinement may actually be somewhat of a novelty and a pleasure. At one time or another we have all wished we could just stay home in bed. Or you may experience a lot of motivation to get those long-awaited projects done. At some point, however, the time ahead of you may begin to seem endless. You may find yourself feeling without interest or goals. At this stage, a daily routine may prove helpful. We are all creatures of habit, more comfortable with a degree of predictability in our lives. Keep in mind, however, that your body and mind may require a little time to adjust to your slower pace. You may find it difficult to concentrate on anything but your body for an extended period of time. Perhaps this is a time to give yourself permission to relax some of those pressures to get things done, and instead do what pleases you and fuels your ability to cope.

It will be a while before a new routine will feel easy and comfortable. You will at first set goals that are too large or too small for your new circumstances. With time you will find a new rhythm—one that allows for rest and self-nurturance as well as for productivity and fun. A sample routine might be as follows:

7 AM   Awaken

            Breakfast

            Read paper *(all of the paper)*

            Nap

10 AM Awaken

Exercise program

Read/television/a project

Noon Lunch

Move to another room or outside

"Chores"/hobbies

Phone call from partner

Nap/relaxation or visualization exercises/practice prepared childbirth breathing

4 PM Exercise program

Shower

Phone call to friend, from friend

6 PM Partner home

Small talk

Watch news

7 PM Dinner

Special time together

Visitors/read/television

10–11 PM Snack

Bed

Of course, your routine will not be ironclad, but some predictable anchor points that are fairly regular will help. Your routine should be as individual as you are, and as flexible as your needs. Establishing it may take some effort, or it may evolve naturally as you pay attention to what feels good during the day. We include a few other general tips derived from experience.

— Set small goals during your day.

— Be flexible about what you want to accomplish. If possible, allow yourself several alternatives for a period of time, to match your interest or energy level. With several alternatives available, you may feel less frustrated when you find you don't have all the tools to do what you had planned.

— If at all possible, have your partner call at a set time each day. It will give you something to look forward to as well as reassuring your partner that you're fine and that there's no cause for worry.

— Take the phone off the hook if you really want to nap or relax.

— Establish something of a weekly routine as well. You may schedule friends or relatives to come on particular days each week to bring lunch or visit. You may schedule your OB visit for the same day each week. Such regularity imparts a rhythm and order similar to that which you normally experience.

— Make it a part of your routine to have some good-quality couple time—time to share your experiences and thoughts, to laugh, and to feel close. Perhaps you can schedule a particular hour each morning or evening to talk to your baby together (encouraging the baby to stay in a little while longer), to feel your baby's movements, to discuss your days, your feelings and frustrations, or just to hold one another. This might be a good time to thank each other for doing so much/so little. Practicing your childbirth education breathing and relaxation techniques or any of the visualization exercises suggested in Chapter Ten can provide a wonderful opportunity for relaxing together and feeling close to one another and your baby.

— Create images that allow you to shift the way you view the premature labor experience, changing images of helplessness and division to perspectives that support the idea of capacity and joint efforts. One couple visualized themselves in a boat in the midst of a swirling storm. There she sat in the bow, big and heavy, holding the compass. And there he was at the stern, small and paddling furiously, providing the necessary movement for their craft. It sometimes felt awkward and unbalanced, but together they were able to keep the boat afloat and to reach their ultimate destination.

Maintaining Your Usual Activities and Roles

As a premature labor patient there is admittedly a lot you can't do. However, there are many things you *can* do that will help you feel you are still capable of making valuable contributions.

If you have worked outside the home, depending upon the type of work, you may be able to continue some projects at home. If you are employed by someone else, a face-to-face meeting at your home may help to convince your employer that you can still carry out some aspects of your job, e.g., daily or weekly visits by co-workers, phone calls, and paperwork. You need to negotiate an understanding concerning what things you can and will do, and those things you can't manage at this time. If you are self-employed, you may have more control. In either case, this may be a time to consider career development: studying that new area, writing that professional paper, reorganizing your resumé.

If you don't work outside the home, or have a job you simply can't do in bed (e.g., outside sales, teaching), there are still many things you can do. The following are some examples:

1. Telephoning to establish your support group.

2. Making arrangements for *anything:* the plumber, the exterminator, the insurance agent, the phone company.

3. Filing for state disability insurance, if eligible.

4. Dealing with medical insurance; you can spend many a happy hour venting your frustrations while figuring out the medical insurance.

5. Arranging for childbirth education. Ask your OB for a list of recommended childbirth educators. While registering for classes (or home instruction, if needed) you can inquire about breastfeeding or childcare classes they might offer. Please refer to Chapter Eight.

6. Calling your hospital to preregister for your delivery, if appropriate in your area.

7. Researching equipment. Ask your friends to pick up copies of baby magazines and local family publications. The ads will give you ideas for shopping by phone or mail. (As you contact people, you'll find that one person can refer another who'll refer another, etc., whom you can contact for items for yourself or baby.)

8. Paying the bills and balancing the checkbook.

9. Taking care of niceties, such as ordering flowers for birthdays, Christmas, Channukah, etc., sending holiday cards, or writing thank-you notes.

10. Planning menus, making grocery lists.

11. Writing in a journal, recording your thoughts and experiences during this challenging part of your life.

Scheduling Support Visits

Often, in our busy lives, we don't have the time to experience just how caring people can be. As you establish your support system, it will be gratifying to realize just how many people you have in your lives who care and will go out of their way to show concern and kindness in a multitude of ways. They will rely upon you, however, for guidance as to just how they can be helpful. One of the best uses of your time can be scheduling other people's volunteer time. As mentioned before, you need to do a little homework and take inventory of just who can do what. You may have dear friends who juggle marriage, children, and work. Obviously their time is at a premium, so just a short social visit would be appropriate. Maybe you could suggest lunch; perhaps order from the takeout place down the street so that they could pick it up on their way. Then there are your relatives or close friends. They desperately want to help, but what to do? Errands! Don't feel shy—give them a list for the market or the drycleaner, ask them to pick up your older child from preschool or water the plants. In this way everyone gets what they want: they're able to make a valuable contribution, the load on your partner is eased, and you can retain a sense of control.

If you don't have family or friends to rely on, or simply don't wish to depend on yours, avail yourselves of the many professional services available. The phone book and local papers are full of cleaning services, errand services, and plant and pet care services. A local church, temple, or community college can be sources for needed support people. Or consider a responsible teenager you know. All of these people are as near as your phone, and you certainly will have the time to interview them. Friends can also be sources for referrals; they may have a cleaning person who has some available time, or who has a friend who would be willing to come to your house and clean. It will take some imagination and determination, but helping people can be found.

With your "found" time, you may be more easily able to show your appreciation than you have been in the past. A short thank-you note for a visit, for a roast brought over, for a chore done, or even for a concerned phone call will make you feel that you're making a small contribution, and will certainly make the giver feel terrific. One pregnant mother scheduled a brunch for a day when she was safely able to get up but before the baby was due, to say thank you to the caretakers who had been especially helpful. This can be a time of more mutual consideration and caring than you have had the opportunity to experience in quite some time.

Now that you have determined who is capable of doing what, you can proceed with scheduling. Scheduling provides several benefits: it ensures that certain things will get done at certain times, it helps pass the time, and it allows you to feel that you're retaining your ability to control your environment.

Scheduling is simply a matter of asking people if they could do certain things at certain times. An example might be:

1. Every other Saturday: cleaning person or a neighborhood teenager dusts, does floors, cleans bathrooms, changes beds, and irons.

2. Every Tuesday and Thursday: Mom and Dad come to bring lunch, water the plants, or do the marketing.

3. Every Wednesday: a relative or close friend brings lunch or a casserole for dinner.

4. A couple of times a week: a friend or friends might come by for a visit or drop by with lunch or dinner.

5. Every Friday: OB visit.

As you can see, a schedule ensures that a lot gets done for the premature labor couple, and it establishes a needed routine as well as helping the time pass. Having a regular schedule of caretakers will limit the number of times you need to find someone to do something at the last minute.

As the Weeks Pass
—Marking Time

Congratulations! Time is passing; your baby is steadily inching toward maturity. You can mark the milestones as major accomplishments for all of you. Most of us, to one degree or another, are goal oriented. One positive thing about premature labor is that thankfully, it is *not* an open-ended proposition. *You have a goal—to get your baby to thirty-seven weeks gesta-*

tion. No matter when you started your period of confinement, you can start the countdown (e.g., twenty-two weeks down, fifteen to go). Pick the day of the week that completes another week passed on the way to your goal, and celebrate! Treat yourself to something special: flowers, a new nightgown, a sip of champagne—and most important, a pat on the back that you each made it through another week.

Keeping track of your baby's development is an especially helpful strategy. Books are a wonderful way of following fetal development, as well as reinforcing the idea that time really *is* passing. One expectant mother established a routine of reading a chapter on her baby's current stage of development and sharing what she had learned with her partner. Books you may find interesting are listed in the Bibliography at the end of this book. As you progress in your pregnancy, you can get books on breastfeeding and childbirth education.

Another way to mark time is, of course, the weekly OB visit. Each visit marks another week passed on the way to your goal. It also provides you with much-needed reassurance regarding your baby's physical well-being as well as your own. Be sure to ask what your baby's weight might be, and your uterine measurement. Many couples keep a list of questions for the visit to be sure their informational needs are met. If your obstetric practitioner seems emotionally accessible, you may choose to share some of your feelings—both fears and triumphs. Your clinician is certainly a central person in your extended support system, and one who is likely to be interested in your complete welfare.

For some couples, the passage of time will signal sufficient progress to warrant occasional extra excursions out of the house. This determination, of course, must be made by your medical practitioner, and must always be undertaken with appropriate attention to the effects of your activity. Added liberties are not only a sign of your progress, they also provide a change of scene that may be just the uplift you and your partner need. Keep in mind that the purpose of getting out is to change your environment, to alleviate boredom, to relax and have fun—it is not intended to make you "keep up" with everyone. You may find that too much animation or excitement may make your uterus irritable and increase your contractions. If this is the case, it is vital that you feel comfortable in saying that you must go home and be quiet.

If you read the previous paragraph with great envy because for you a more conservative treatment is necessary, establish some changes of scenery within your own home; move into another room, or outside. Bring the change of social scenery to you. With attention to your activity and excitement level, there is no reason why you can't have a potluck dinner party, for example.

As your pregnancy progresses, you and your partner may wish to attend childbirth, childcare, or breastfeeding classes. Chapter Eight addresses childbirth education more fully, including issues related to premature labor. Aside from their obvious informational value, these classes can provide a needed change of scene and an opportunity to talk with other pregnant couples. As in other social situations, lie down (please don't feel the need to apologize) and listen to your body. If you feel an increase in contractions, it is time to call it a day, go home and rest. For the homebound couple, there are cassettes and films on childbirth and childcare topics that you may be able to rent. In addition, many childbirth instructors will come to your home and give you a "mini" course in prepared childbirth. Check with a childbirth instructor, or your local childbirth education associations or library.

Preparing for the baby. Part of the excitement of a pregnancy is, of course, planning for the arrival of your baby. As discussed in Chapter Two, some couples experiencing premature labor temporarily put a lid on their anticipation of the birth because of their fears for the baby's health or survival. Making plans and purchases, however, is an important part of the "nesting" process and of beginning to bond with your baby. It is also an important way for couples to deal with the long waiting period of pregnancy.

As the weeks pass, you will probably want to make plans for your baby's arrival. You will be wondering what type of equipment to buy, and where. You may want to decorate a nursery or plan some space that will accommodate and welcome your child. We encourage you to do so both as a means of feeling your optimism and excitement about your baby, and as a way of spending some joyful time together.

It is certainly true that "the best crib you can give your baby is your uterus"—for now. Because you are in bed doing so, however, you may fear that you will be cheated out of the fun of shopping for and decorating an external home for your child. What follows are some suggestions for doing just that from your bedside.

1. *Layette*

Friends with children, magazines, or your own experience can give you an idea of what you may want. Layette items are easily listed for family members or friends to pick up for you. Watch for advertised sales at major department stores, which can offer extremely good prices. Many parents' publications list mail-order sources of unique clothing and natural fibers. Write for information and get yourself put on some mailing lists.

2. *Baby 'Paraphernalia'*

Diapers, baby lotion, Q-tips, Desitin, and other supplies are all important for the nursery. Again, you can give a list to one of the prospective grand-parents, godparents, or aunts/uncles, and they'll have great fun; or you may want to wait until you're up and able to get these things yourself.

3. *Furniture and Equipment*

This gets a little trickier, but it can be done. Have members of your support system shop baby stores and bring you catalogues or pamphlets for bassinets, cribs, changing tables, and dressers. Alternatively, you can call or write to request brochures and catalogues. The Yellow Pages will list stores in your area as well as specialty shops. Your local childbirth educa-tion and La Leche League chapters may also know of supply outlets for mother and infant equipment.

4. *The Room*

You can, if you like, arrange to have your nursery painted or wallpapered professionally. Some local artists will do custom murals. Check the Yellow Pages or local baby publications. Most arrangements can be made by phone, as many decorator centers offer "shop-at-home" services. Many shops will loan wallpaper books for you to take home. Alternatively, you can arrange a "paint the nursery" party—invite friends, and provide the food and paint brushes! An expectant mother can supervise or check the progress of the painting on her bathroom stops (which will probably for unmentioned reasons be more frequent that day).

The important thing to keep in mind is that your newborn's needs are very, very simple. If you wish to outfit your nursery before your baby's birth, you're limited only by your imagination. On the other hand if you choose to wait, be assured that nourishment, a couple of nighties, diapers, and lots of love are all your baby needs to feel welcomed to this world.

5. *The Baby Shower*

If you have an established circle of friends and family in the area, someone may want to give you a baby shower. If you and your clinician agree that a shower would be fine, lie down, hold court, and enjoy! However, if you or your obstetrical practitioner feel that the excitement may have an adverse effect on your irritable uterus, have the shower after the baby has been born and you have had an opportunity to settle in (perhaps six or eight weeks). It's a perfect opportunity for everyone to see the baby and celebrate your accomplishment.

We hope you feel encouraged to shop at home and to proceed with many of the exciting aspects of pregnancy. Over the course of your bedrest experience, you will weave in and out of different attitudes toward time. At times you will appreciate the luxury of delving into a sedentary project in depth, and time will seem to fly. At other times (probably when you feel less encouraged or toward the middle of your weeks in bed), you may swear that time has stopped. Some self-management, as we've suggested, will help. In general, however, your perceptions of time probably reflect your feelings in the areas described in Chapter Two. When time seems to drag, some reflection on what you're feeling, in conjunction with the practical modifications we've suggested here, may provide relief.

TIME PRESSURE

> *I don't even have a child yet, but I feel like a single parent!*
>
> *Expectant Father*

As the partner of a premature labor patient, you find yourself quite suddenly with too much to do and too little time in which to do it. You will probably feel stressed, tired, frustrated, resentful of all this responsibility, and perhaps envious of the fact that your partner seems to have all the time in the world with nothing to do. You may also feel guilty about feeling this resentment and envy. You feel continual time pressure: the sense that the time in which you must accomplish numerous things is too short.

A certain amount of time pressure can be catalyzing. As you've probably experienced in other contexts, a deadline can provide the extra push to get a job done. What must be acknowledged in addition is that each of us has our own threshold, after which time pressures become stressful and lead to dysfunctional anxiety. Signs that one has crossed this line include the feeling that something must be done before a deadline, or that time is "running out" and that something terrible will happen when it does.

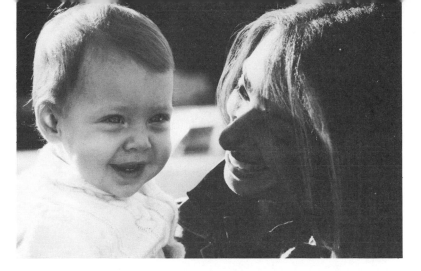

Elysa Waldholz-Goldblatt (fashion-buyer) and daughter Jamie (age one year). Jamie was born at term after Elysa's preterm labor was diagnosed at thirty-four weeks of pregnancy. She was treated with bedrest and medication. *Credit: Hella Hammid*

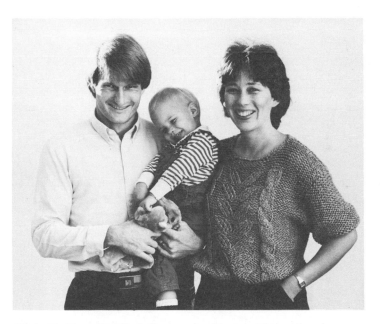

Cindy P. Gates (medical illustrator) with son Christopher (age two years) and husband William. Christopher was born at thirty-three weeks of gestation after Cindy's pregnancy was complicated by both a weakened cervix and premature labor. Cindy was on bedrest for twenty weeks during her pregnancy. *Credit: Hella Hammid*

Joe Landon (writer) and daughter Emily (age three months). Emily was born at term, after Joe's wife Laura had spent sixteen weeks on complete bedrest for premature labor. During this time of bedrest, Emily's brother Aaron was two years old. *Credit: Hella Hammid*

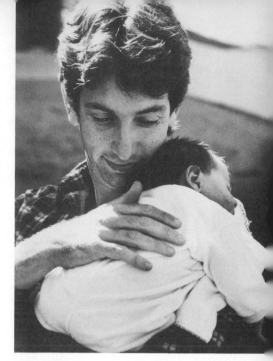

Sara Davidson (author) with children Rachel (age five months) and Andrew (age two and a half years). Rachel and Andrew were both born at term after complicated pregnancies, each requiring twenty-four weeks of bedrest during the pregnancy. *Credit: Hella Hammid*

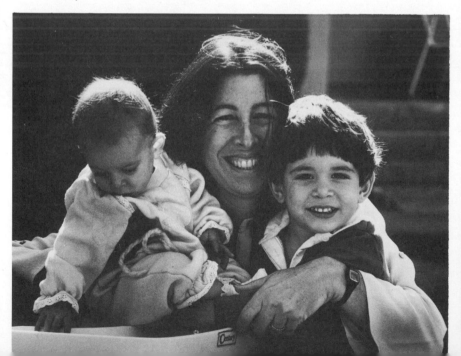

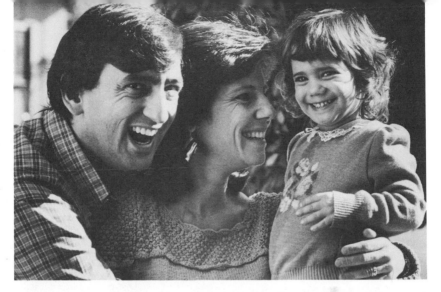

Bonnie Ziveta Silverman (social worker) with daughter Rachel (age three years) and husband Daniel. Rachel was born at thirty-seven weeks of gestation after Bonnie's pregnancy was complicated with premature labor and high blood pressure. *Credit: Hella Hammid*

Laura Landon (homemaker) with son Aaron (age two years). Laura was on bedrest for over three months while pregnant with her daughter Emily while Aaron was an active toddler. She was able to find creative approaches to mothering Aaron while on bedrest. *Credit: Hella Hammid*

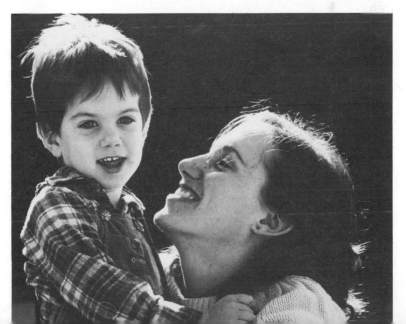

Florence G. Blatt with grand-daughter Jamie (age one year). Florence was separated geographically from her daughter Elysa during Elysa's month of bedrest for premature labor, which she found very difficult as a mother and expectant grandmother. *Credit: Elysa Waldholz-Goldblatt*

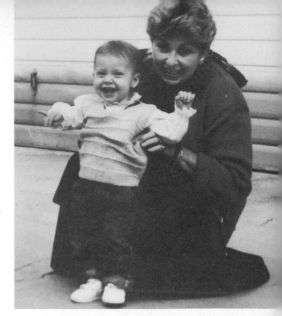

Marsha Kinder Bautista (professor) with children Gabriela (age twelve years), Victor (age eighteen months), and husband Nicolás. Victor was born at twenty-eight weeks of gestation after Marsha had undergone bedrest throughout her pregnancy, which was complicated with uterine fibroids, vaginal bleeding, a weakened cervix (a cerclage was placed), and premature labor (she received medication). *Credit: Hella Hammid*

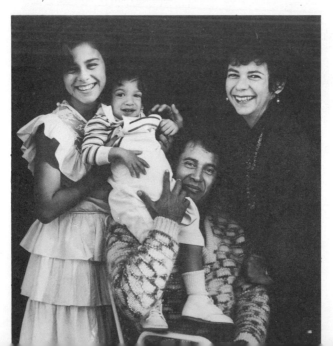

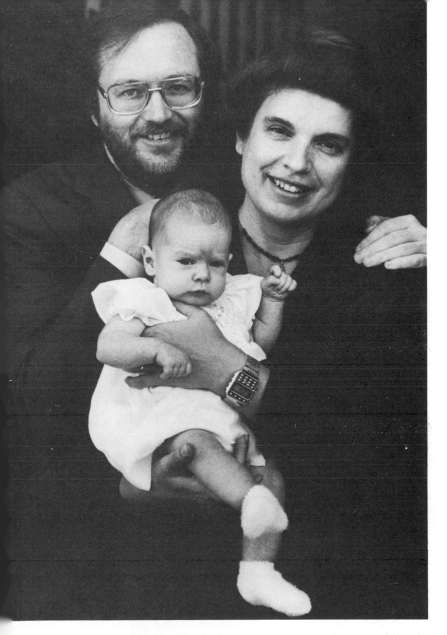

Britta Lindgren (aerospace engineer) with partner Kevin Savage and daughter Ciren (age two months). Britta had premature labor diagnosed at thirty-two weeks of pregnancy, which was treated with five weeks of bedrest. *Credit: Hella Ham mid*

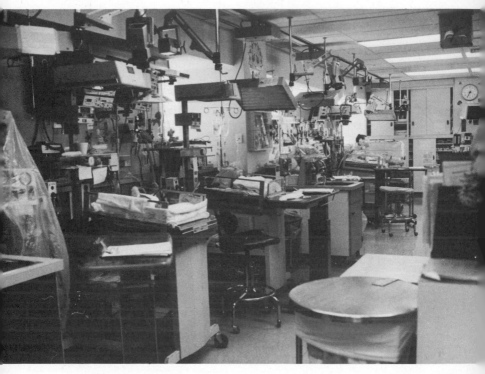

Neonatal Intensive Care Unit at the University of California at Los Angeles Medical Center.   *Credit: Hella Hammid*

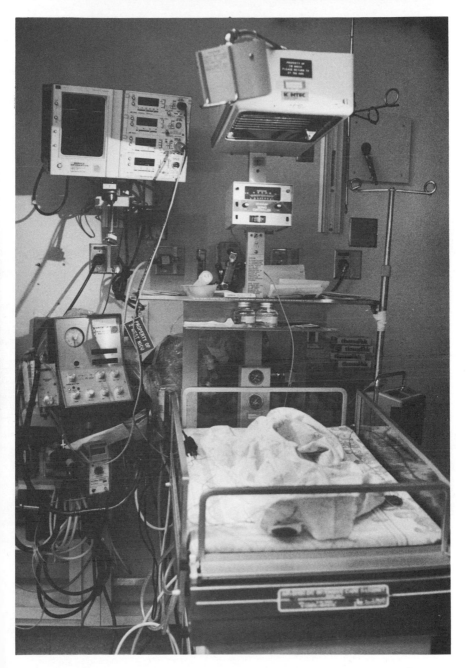

Medical equipment involved in the care of a premature baby.   *Credit: Hella Hammid*

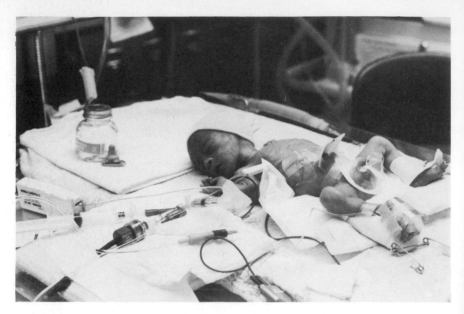

Premature baby in Neonatal Intensive Care Unit. *Credit: Linda McKirdy, R.N.*

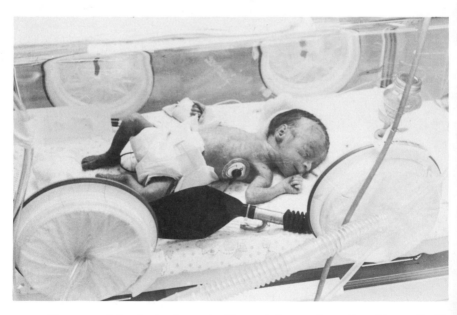

Premature baby in incubator in Neonatal Intermediate Care Unit. *Credit: Linda McKirdy, R.N.*

Friedman and Rosenman[2] call this "hurry sickness." As the partner of a woman in premature labor, you may at least from time to time have "hurry sickness." Contributing to it are both the realities of your sudden responsibility for additional tasks and your own thoughts about your responsibilities and pressures. We will consider practical ways to delegate and limit your responsibilities, as well as offer hints for modifying the way you think about your time pressures.

Antidotes For Time Pressure
(adapted from the above-cited Friedman and Rosenman, 1974):

— Each day remind yourself that life is a process. This period in time *will* give way to the next. In so doing, it is most important to preserve that which will have some continuity. Time spent nurturing your relationship with your partner may in the long run be more productive than sweeping the cobwebs from the corner. On the other hand, there may be times when sweeping the cobwebs from the corner is what your partner needs to feel nurtured. In short, when confronted with multiple pressures, ask yourself, "Will this be important five years from now?" and "Must I act now, or can something else take precedence?"

— Avoid thinking about many things at the same time. When your "to do" list keeps intruding, write it down. Constant vigilant thinking about what you have to do is sometimes a way of rehearsing so that you won't forget. By writing things down, you can set priorities, and then table the less important details.

— Give yourself an elastic time schedule whenever you can. This may need to be negotiated with your partner, who in all probability will look forward to your arrival home at the appointed hour. Make clear what your mutual needs are to avoid disappointment.

— Consider the *value* of your time. Do you really want to give up X amount of time for X amount of money or other payoff?

— Avoid projecting time pressure onto others. You may feel that others, especially your partner, expect a certain amount of things to be done by a certain time. In reality, the other person may

---

2. Friedman, Meyer, and Rosenman, Ray H. *Type A Behavior and Your Heart.* New York: Fawcett Crest, 1974.

have no such expectations, or a different set of expectations. Talk about it.

— Take breaks in the midst of any activity, long or short, that may be stress-producing. Sometimes we charge full steam ahead with the aim of getting finished no matter what. When finally finished, we've worked ourselves into such a frazzle that completion holds no reward save exhaustion and frenzy. A break may restore perspective and calm.

— Find periods each day for relaxation, visualization, and/or exercise.

The goal of relieving time pressure is to free you from the anxiety that binds and drains your energy. Once this perceived time pressure is eased, you may be able to consider some time-saving strategies.

Set daily goals and *establish priorities* for them. When Charles Schwab was president of Bethlehem Steel, he asked a consultant for advice about how to make better use of his time. The consultant suggested he write down the six most important tasks he had to do each day, and to rank order their importance. The consultant added, "Don't worry if you only finish one or two. If you can't finish them all by this method, you couldn't by any other method either. At least this way you'll know which ones are most important." Several weeks later Mr. Schwab sent the consultant a check for $25,000, with a note saying that it was the most profitable advice he'd ever received!

Initially, setting priorities for household chores and responsibilities needs to be a process shared with your partner. Negotiate what is truly most important to each of you to preserve your senses of orderliness, convenience, and control. Decide what you can let slide. Accept the fact that things will not be done exactly as before. Negotiating with explicitness about what is acceptable to each of you can prevent projection, resentment, and disappointment.

As the premature labor patient, you will have to abdicate your responsibility concerning physical household duties. On your way to the bathroom you may notice dustballs the size of tumbleweed on the floor, or three days' worth of dishes on the sink. Close your eyes, grit your teeth, and keep walking. When it comes right down to it, dustballs and dishes are just not worth an argument or bad feelings.

As the partner of a premature labor patient, you'll have to get used to either absorbing the responsibilities formerly undertaken by your partner, delegating them, or doing without. Earlier in this chapter and in previous chapters we discussed the need to rely on others when possible. Your contract with your partner may include agreements about who will ask whom to do what to help out. Your mutually established priorities will go a long way toward creating a new order. However, it will take some trial and error and renegotiating before you arrive at what's really important—and what's important today may not be so tomorrow. Try to remember how vulnerable your partner feels, especially physically. She'll feel that not only is her life out of control, but her body too. It is therefore especially important that mutually agreed-upon responsibilities be fulfilled or renegotiated —it will provide both of you with a sense of control, as well as continuing to cement your partnership during this difficult time.

Other Time Savers

— Capitalize on your prime time. When during the day are you at your best for certain tasks? Try to schedule yourself accordingly, to make the most of the interaction between your body clock and the time clock.

— Make the most of already committed time (e.g., waiting-room time, commuting time) with reading materials, a tape recorder, and a pad available for making lists or jotting down spontaneous ideas.

— Schedule some quiet time each day to work alone, reflect on the day before, and be with your own thoughts.

We can't emphasize enough the importance of personal time for the partner of a woman in premature labor. It becomes easy to feel like the supporter only, with you yourself lost somewhere amidst the many demands for your time and attention. It becomes critical to rediscover yourself, to identify your own needs for support and nurturance, and to act to fulfill them. You are not unlike the marathon runner who must establish a reasonable pace, or spend your energy too quickly. Being that runner in the best sense, you can use this process to become sensitively attuned to your own body and psyche if you pay attention and honor it.

SPACE

Once a diagnosis of premature labor is made, the challenge of providing for the woman's physical needs for comfort and quietude emerges. In so doing, you will need to establish what we refer to as "nests." This refers to the two or three locations you will construct as your sites for repose, stocked with "essentials" for comfort, entertainment, and nourishment.

We suggest that you pick *several* places in your home in which you can comfortably nest. For example, you may have one nest in your bedroom, another in your living room or den, and another outside (if weather permits). Once established, these bases give you alternatives in scenery to choose from after each bathroom stop.

We suggest that *each nest* be equipped with the following on a permanent basis, so that when you want a change of scene it's a simple matter of walking, and not of moving the entire nest:

1. Place to stretch out: bed, chaise, or couch.

2. Cinder blocks: to prop up the foot of the bed or couch in Trendelenburg position if advised by your medical practitioner.

3. Eggcrate mattress: a foam pad designed to distribute your weight more evenly, preventing sores and back pain. This mattress is available through your hospital or medical supply rental companies. Prices can vary, so you may want to shop by phone before purchasing. (In most cases, your medical insurance will cover at least part of the cost. If not, save the receipt for income-tax purposes.) You will need the eggcrate mattress only at your primary nest, probably where you sleep through the night.

4. Lots of pillows, pretty sheets, and cases. Acquiring these is a great errand for someone in your support system. They needn't be expensive; check local discount stores.

5. A chair for visitors.

Please remember that it's not necessary to have all of these things; however, they may provide a more comfortable environment for you.

The next list includes items that you *may* want to have at one location or at each nest, or to put in a tote bag that you can carry to each nest when you wish to move:

1. TV, *TV Guide*, remote control. You may watch more TV now than you've ever watched in your life! You might want to consider investing temporarily in cable with the movie options.

2. Radio or cassette recorder.

3. A mobile telephone. This is a great investment, available in a variety of stores; check for the best prices. This phone will also come in handy when you are breastfeeding or following a toddler around. (Don't forget the phone book.)

4. Alarm clock. This will be essential to remind you to take your medication, if prescribed, especially during the night. Programmable clocks allow you to set the alarm for up to three separate times before falling asleep. This will save you from having to rely on your sleepy memory to reset the clock in the middle of the night.

5. An extra prescription of your medication, e.g., Ritodrine or Terbutaline. Nothing is worse than running out of your pills and panicking about how to get a refill. It is also a good idea to shop around (by phone) for the best price, and then inform the pharmacist that you'll need it for the next several months so the pharmacy will be sure to stock it. Find one that delivers.

6. An "Able Table": a table that fits over your thighs, can be raised to accommodate your growing uterus, tilts to a variety of positions, and has a catch rim to hold paper, books, pencils, and pens. It's available at medical supply rental companies. This will enable you to do paperwork, crafts, or hobbies at an angle.

7. A pregnancy wedge. As mentioned in Chapter One, this is a wedge that fits under your belly for support when you are lying on your side. It has a machine-washable cover, and is available from:

> Body Therapeutics
> 6317 Wilshire Boulevard #503
> Los Angeles, CA 90048
> (213) 655-6021

8. Liquid antacid. Many practitioners suggest an antacid to ease the indigestion caused by lying down to eat. Discuss this possibility with your clinician.

9. Kleenex. Lying with your feet higher than your head may cause a stuffy nose.

10. Chapstick. You may get chapped lips from breathing through your mouth.

11. Piles of books and magazines. If you have friends with small children, ask them to save their issues of parenting publications—full of useful information, ideas, and things to send for.

12. A cooler or collection of nonperishable snacks/drinks. If your kitchen and refrigerator are not convenient to a "bathroom run," you'll have to keep your lunch and snacks by each nest.

13. Handicrafts, hobbies, paperwork.

14. Paper, pencils, stationery.

15. A mirror, comb, brush, cosmetics for primping.

16. Inflatable shampoo basin. If you find yourself needing to shampoo in bed, this inflatable basin allows you to do so. It has a drain table for changing water and edging to protect your bed linens. Available from:

> Comfortably Yours
> 52 West Hunter Avenue
> Maywood, NJ 07607
> (201) 368-0400

Whew, you say! Where will all that fit? In piles here and stacks there . . . under your night stand . . . on your partner's pillow . . . under the TV stand, so you can grab it on the way back from the bathroom. Your nest areas are bound to look more or less like organized (or disorganized) chaos. Periodically it will drive you nuts, and then you will "spring clean" (by directing someone else, please).

Because you have to live with so many things within rolling distance, it is important to pay as much attention as possible to the other aesthetics of your "nest" sites. Choose locations that offer a lot of light, both natural and artificial. Accept graciously all offers of plants and flowers. If your home is large, choose locations that avoid stairs. Choose at least one location that allows you to see what's happening on the street, should you choose to watch the world continuing to function as usual.

Being alone in a house, especially when you feel physically vulnerable, can for some people raise concerns about what to do in an emergency. Of course, nothing is likely to happen, but you may feel more secure if you take a few precautions. Be sure your smoke alarms work. Be sure several neighbors know of your situation. (Busybody neighbors are the best for this sort of thing, as they will be sure to notice anything unusual.) Give keys to people who will be coming regularly (including a neighbor). Ask all visitors to notify you before they come, so you can arrange to keep the doors locked otherwise. Keep a list of emergency numbers at your bedside. If you do have an emergency and need to call an ambulance for transportation rather than waiting for your partner or a neighbor, be sure the ambulance will take you to the hospital where you expect to deliver. Some paramedic ambulances will take you only to the officially designated hospital, which may be different from the one where your obstetrician practices. If you have a plan for handling an emergency, you will be better able to set aside any worries you might have.

We hope this chapter has been of some help with the "how-to's" of your premature labor experience. Please remember, these ideas have been compiled from the experience of former premature labor patients. Some may be useful, some not—use this chapter for your reference.

We would like to end this chapter with some memories from former premature labor patients. Some of them may strike a familiar chord, or at least conjure up a humorous image.

— Thirteen weeks of crumbs in the bed.

— The nurse who woke me up to tell me I'd have to take a pill in half an hour.

— Being "on hold."

— Spaghetti sauce on the sheets.

— Needing to ask someone to run water in the nearby sink so that the sound would stimulate my success in using the bed pan.

— Planning my escape route in case a madman broke into the house.

— Aunt Sarah's apple surprise!

— Orgasms in my sleep, for lack of them at any other time (a little worry, a lot of relief).

— When did the baby last move?

— More spaghetti sauce on the sheets.

— Itchy support hose. (Maybe it would help if my legs could be shaved!)

— Shaving my partner's legs for her. (This is intimacy?)

— Come to your house to cut your hair? Sure! Call me again in about a month. Then I should be in a better personal space.

— More crumbs in the bed.

— What week is this?

THE HOSPITAL EXPERIENCE

*by Mary Sue Ulven, R.N., and
Patricia Robertson, M.D.*

> *"Go to the hospital? To labor and delivery? But it's not
> time yet to have this baby."*

Complicated pregnancy situations involving premature labor and/or weakened cervix may require hospitalization, which often includes medications and/or surgery. Hospitalization is usually a very foreign concept to the pregnant woman and her partner, who had only considered going to the hospital near the time of the due date for a normal birth. This chapter discusses hospitalization and how to cope with it.

REASONS FOR HOSPITALIZATION

To be told to go to the hospital Labor and Delivery Unit, when your due date is still far off, is quite a shock. Until recently, you and your partner had expected the hospital experience to be a brief and singular one, occurring at the end of the pregnancy. To be hospitalized earlier is usually an unexpected and frightening experience. Hospitals, by their very nature, are intimidating places, usually associated with illness, not health. For the average woman in this situation, it may be the first time she has ever been hospitalized. Few young, healthy couples are familiar with the complexity of the hospital environment. Specialized routines, complex procedures, sterile surroundings, and numerous personnel often blend to create a seemingly strange place. Medical terminology can even sound like a foreign language, and may be incomprehensible to anxious, prospective parents. Coping with all of the various aspects of hospitalization is difficult, and often serves only to bewilder and frustrate the woman and her partner.

The strong emotions accompanying this situation can further complicate coping ability. Fear, anxiety, confusion, frustration, guilt, anger, loss —all are common emotional reactions to preterm labor and subsequent hospitalization. There may be feelings of loss of control over a precious and personal event in your lives. Hospital personnel and routines seem to take over; the pregnant woman is poked and prodded, subjected to numerous tests and procedures, and must even succumb to hospital regimentation as to when she can eat and sleep. Her partner may feel left out, unable to support and care for her in these disturbing circumstances.

However, the hospital experience does not need to be a negative one. Knowledge about hospital routines and procedures, about what to expect and how to cope, puts you and your partner back in control. While the experience may still be a difficult one, the couple who is informed and involved will ultimately gain strength from it. Knowledge of common procedures and routines will lessen your apprehensions and also enable you to communicate better with your doctor and the hospital personnel; you then become involved in your own health care. This knowledge and involvement not only decreases your anxiety, but ultimately improves your health care.

"Why do I need to be hospitalized?" This may be your first question. The woman experiencing signs of premature labor or weakened cervix usually still feels and looks healthy; she may not even have been aware of the premature contractions or weakening cervix until informed by her obstetrical practitioner. The minor symptoms may not seem to you or your partner to require hospitalization. It is hard to believe the situation is so serious. After all, you don't feel sick! And in truth, you are not really ill. However, because the uterus is contracting or the cervix is weakening, the possibility of premature birth for your baby is quite real. If premature labor or weakened cervix is not detected and stopped in the very early stages, premature delivery will usually result. Early, conservative treatment is the best guarantee against early delivery.

The hospital provides the trained personnel and technology needed to treat preterm labor and ensure the well-being of both mother and baby. Not all women who are admitted to Labor and Delivery are there to deliver; they may be there to prevent delivery. Few hospitals have special units for high-risk antepartum women; instead, these women are usually admitted to the Labor and Delivery Unit, which can provide the intensive observation and care that is initially required in these situations. Because often there is not a separate area for the care of prenatal patients, a laboring mother may be in the next room in the Labor and Delivery Suite. This exposure to someone laboring next door may be positive, enabling you to focus on the endpoint of your pregnancy, but it may also be distracting, especially if a lot of noise accompanies the labor. It is often disconcerting and even frightening to hear other women who are not coping well with their labor. You may overhear a conversation about problem deliveries. Such negative input can easily cast a shadow over the anticipation of your own labor and delivery. Don't hold back your questions, concerns, and feelings about what you are hearing. Ask your nurse. The other side of the picture may reveal a different perspective. Remember, too, that you are not hearing all the other women who are well prepared for birth and are coping without making noise.

Once the preterm labor is stable, you will probably be transferred from the Labor and Delivery Unit to a room on the maternity floor in a quieter environment with another preterm labor patient as your roommate, or to a private room. Once you have been stabilized, you can usually go home in a few days.

A hospital stay is rarely expected or desired, but it is often the best place for the close observation necessary to determine the specific treatment plan that the woman with preterm labor or a weakened cervix needs. Your best key to coping with the hospitalization is to stay involved and informed.

THE HOSPITAL ROUTINE

Admission

On admission to the hospital, you are usually taken to the Labor and Delivery Suite. There you will meet your nurse, who will orient you to your room. The first event is to change from your clothes into a hospital gown. (You can keep your underwear on if you like.) A urine sample is usually obtained as a "midstream clean catch" to rule out any bladder infection.

When you are settled in bed (usually in the Trendelenburg position), two external monitor belts are applied to your abdomen. The first belt is to detect any premature labor contractions, and the second is to measure the heart beat of the baby. Once the well-being of the fetus has been assured, the belt recording the fetal heartbeat is often removed and only the uterine contraction belt kept in place. It is very important that the uterine contraction belt is below your navel. If the monitor does not seem to be showing contractions, even though you can feel them, be sure to tell your nurse. While the initial monitoring is being recorded, blood samples are often drawn to check for any infection or anemia (CBC). Occasionally, clotting studies are obtained to rule out any premature placental separation (DIC screen). Sometimes an ultrasound examination is done to determine additional factors involved in possible preterm labor or weakened cervix.

A vaginal examination is usually then done by your obstetrician, if it was not done that day in the office. The vaginal examination may have two parts: checking to be sure that no amniotic fluid is leaking, and checking the five different cervical parameters to assess the status of the cervix. This cervical examination will usually be repeated at intervals during your hospital stay to be sure that the cervix is responding to the treatment. However, if amniotic fluid is leaking, these exams in most cases are eliminated in order to avoid possible infection, and other parameters are used for treatment decisions.

Once a plan has been devised to treat your preterm labor or weakened cervix, its various parts will be put into effect by the nurse. The usual plan involves bedrest (ask your nurse to order you an eggcrate mattress to decrease the hardness of the hospital bed during a prolonged stay), hydration, and often medication. Please see Appendix B on medical procedures for a detailed discussion of vaginal examinations, ultrasound, monitoring, and cultures.

Nurses

Many people are surprised by the great division of labor in hospitals; sometimes it seems that there is a different person for each task. The one staff person with whom you will interact most frequently is your nurse. Doctors' busy schedules prevent them from being readily available to you at all times during your hospitalization, unless your situation is critical. Usually you will see your doctor at least once a day, and occasionally more often, if necessary. Your nurse, however, is more accessible and is quite familiar with your treatment plan. You will see your nurse frequently, and of course, the nursing staff will be continually accessible to you should you need assistance more frequently. The nurse is responsible for coordinating and carrying out the different aspects of your care, and will be in regular communication with your doctor.

Most hospitals divide the 24 hours of the day into three eight-hour nursing shifts (7 A.M. to 3 P.M., 3 P.M. to 11 P.M., 11 P.M. to 7 A.M.). Some hospitals have 12-hour nursing shifts (7 A.M. to 7 P.M., 7 P.M. to 7 A.M.). This division means that on each shift you will be assigned a different nurse who will be responsible for your care. You will meet your nurse at the beginning of the shift. Remember this person and establish a rapport. For the next eight to twelve hours, while a variety of faces pass by performing various tests and procedures, your nurse may be the only person you see consistently. The familiarity of one person amidst the sea of faces can be comforting and reassuring. If you are hospitalized for several days, you may be assigned the same "evening" nurse, "day" nurse, and "night" nurse so that you can establish some continuity. Requesting this assignment may help you feel more at home. On the other hand, by meeting all the different labor and delivery nurses, you may be more comfortable when you ultimately return for your labor and delivery experience.

Utilizing a holistic approach to patient care, nurses try to see that the needs of the whole person are met. Nursing functions range from providing basic comfort measures, such as personal hygiene, to full assessment of your response to treatment. Besides adjusting and interpreting the monitor and administering medications, your nurse can provide information and clarify misunderstandings. Most nurses realize that small gestures and basic comforts often mean as much to the expectant mother and her partner as does the complicated technology that is ensuring the baby's welfare. Many nurses see themselves as patient advocates, helping to keep you informed and in communication with your doctor. Be assured that your nurse is genuinely concerned for your welfare, both physical and psychological. Take advantage of this knowledge and caring. Your nurse can be a valuable resource person, available to answer your questions, explain hospital routines and procedures, offer reassurance and support, and suggest ways to increase your comfort.

Visitors

Hospitals must necessarily place some limitation on visitors. A family-oriented maternity department, however, will often have its own visiting policies. Maternity visitor restrictions have been relaxed in recent years as the value of family support has gained recognition.

Both you and your partner are concerned and anxious about what this hospitalization means. Staying together physically will enable you to support each other. Most maternity departments will allow your partner to stay with you much of the time. If you're in a private room, your partner may even be able to stay overnight on a cot. If you have other children, ask if there are special visiting hours for them. If not, see if special arrangements can be made; it is important for you to see each other at this time.

When anticipating other visitors, consider how you feel, whom you want to see, and what effect they will have on you. Visitors may prove more tiring than you expect. Someone who makes you tense may trigger some contractions. Many women hospitalized for preterm labor discover that they must limit visitors and phone calls if they are to have any time to rest. Consider scheduling your visitors, so that you are not overwhelmed by too many people at once. Discuss your concerns with your nurse. If you don't want to offend your well-meaning but tiring friends and relatives, ask your nurse to monitor your visitors and to impose restrictions (e.g., limit each visitor to fifteen minutes). See if you can restrict incoming phone calls. Calm, uninterrupted periods of time are important for you, both physically and emotionally.

On the other hand, visitors may be a cheerful highlight in an otherwise boring day. Capitalize on their concern for you. When they ask what they can do for you, tell them! Perhaps they can run an errand for you, relieving your partner of an extra chore. Ask them to bring food, books, magazines, a TV guide—whatever you would like that isn't available.

Spend some time now thinking about your feelings about visitors—what will work out best for you, your partner, and your baby?

Sleeping

Hospitals are not always the best place to get some rest. Activities continue around the clock. Walls are not soundproofed. Many women in preterm labor are awakened frequently for medications. Some of these medications may interfere with your ability to sleep well; others may knock you out in the middle of the day. Nurses are in and out of your room frequently to check the monitor. Such chaos in your sleep schedule can lead to feelings of disorientation and produce difficulty in coping.

Carefully consider your needs, and communicate them to your health caretakers. With planning, you may be able to adapt the hospital schedule to one which works better for you. Below is a list of options for your reflection. Would they help you to cope better? If so, is the nursing staff amenable to them?

Private rooms provide a much better atmosphere for rest. Is one available for you? If not, ask if your roommate could be another preterm labor patient who has similar needs.

The average hospital day begins at 7 A.M., with breakfast then or shortly thereafter. Request a cold breakfast, so that you may sleep later and eat at your leisure.

Schedule your visitors. If visiting hours are lenient, ask relatives and friends to call before they come to visit.

Ask that phone calls be intercepted when you are resting. If this is not possible, take the phone off the hook.

Request that your partner be provided with a cot or comfortable lounge chair so that important sleep or rest is available for both of you.

Eating

Hospital food has long been the object of many jokes. In various hospitals, it ranges from inedible to surprisingly agreeable. Initially, until your condition is assessed as stable, you may not be allowed to eat. Your doctor may want you "NPO"—taking nothing by mouth. Or you may be restricted to clear fluids only.

When you are allowed to eat a regular diet, the hospital's menu and meal schedule may prove exasperating. The food selections can quickly become boring. You may find that the three scheduled eating times are inappropriate for you; many pregnant women prefer to eat smaller meals more frequently. When you are restricted to bedrest, digestion is further hampered by the Trendelenburg position. Heartburn is often more frequent in this position. Ask your doctor for a liquid antacid if this is a problem for you.

Women who are vegetarians or who follow restricted diets for medical or religious reasons may find their menu choices dismally meager. You need not resign yourself to the dictates of the hospital dietary department. This is one area where you can take more control. Your nurse may be a good person to ask about possible options, or you can talk with the hospital dietitian. Obtain the following information and consider how you can best meet your dietary needs and desires.

What is readily available to you on the unit—juices, jello, custard, crackers?

Can you have snacks delivered to you between meals (or stored in the refrigerator until you want them)? Can you order anything that is not on the menu?

If nothing on the menu appeals to you, can you somehow get a voucher for food from the employee cafeteria?

Can your partner, friends, or relatives bring you meals?

Is there a refrigerator on the unit where you can keep a small supply of your own favorite foods?

Is there a microwave oven on the unit that could be used to heat or reheat meals you slept through or food brought in to you?

Are there any good takeout restaurants near the hospital? Perhaps your partner can bring in food from them for both of you.

Transfer to the Postpartum Unit

Once your contractions are stopped or are well under control, you may no longer need the intensive care and observation offered by the labor and delivery nurses. As a safeguard, your doctor may want you to stay in the hospital, but without the constant monitoring. At this point, you may be transferred from labor and delivery to the postpartum (already delivered) unit, which often includes antepartum (undelivered) patients as well.

Postpartum nurses have a greater number of patients to care for, so you may not be as familiar with them as you are with the labor and delivery nurses. However, after several days on the floor, you will probably know them well. On the postpartum floor, the monitoring is not as intense as in labor and delivery, allowing for longer rest periods. Take advantage of these rest periods, when someone other than yourself can make sure you get your medication on time!

Preparing for Hospital Discharge

Once you have been discharged from the hospital, you will be having regular office visits. On the day of your discharge, be sure that you understand the plan for the home front. Make certain that you have the appropriate medications if applicable (medications to stop the premature labor contractions, stool softener, iron pills, etc.). Be sure that your activity instructions are clear. Be certain that you know when your practitioner wants to be informed of the level of contractions, if in fact it seems that things are getting out of control. If you have some difficulty in planning your discharge (whether to your home or to the home of a family member), remember that there is usually a social worker available in the hospital to let you know about community resources that might help you as part of your home treatment. Although usually only one hospitalization is necessary for treatment of preterm labor or a weakened cervix, a small percentage of women in preterm labor may need multiple hospitalizations.

No one wants to be hospitalized, but you may find it is not as bad as you expected. There is also a positive side to it, which you may want to emphasize to yourself: You are now familiar with all the hospital policies and routines, and you know many of the nurses. For couples who find themselves in and out of the hospital, the nursing staff often becomes another source of support. When you come back for the delivery, familiarity will put you more at ease. If the baby does arrive early, you will already be aware of how to cope with hospitalization and to whom to go for answers and support. More likely, you will return to deliver a full-term baby and the whole staff will rejoice with you.

COPING PSYCHOLOGICALLY WITH HOSPITALIZATION

Preterm labor in itself is a great stress; hospitalization for preterm labor further exacerbates the difficulties. As we have continually emphasized in this book, a major key to coping is being informed and involved in your own care. Don't let the hospital and its routines turn you into a passive patient. Assert your individuality. Use the information in this chapter to increase your and your partner's involvement in your care.

Create your own space in the hospital environment. Although you may not have much physical space, make what there is your own. Organize it so that you know where your belongings are. Have your partner's chair strategically located. Have some personal items brought in from your home—pillows with colored cases, pictures of other children or a favorite vacation spot, your own nightgown, a radio cassette player. These personal items reinforce the feeling that this is your space. Having your own space fulfills a deep need, creating stability amid the hospital chaos and providing comfort and security.

Don't feel that you need to ask the nurse for every little thing. Have your partner help you with bathing, brushing your teeth, and using the bed pan if needed. Ask your nurse to show your partner where items such as ice water, juice, and extra blankets are located. Assisting you will help your mate feel of more value.

The partner of the hospitalized woman may feel intimidated by the hospital environment. Your involvement is a valuable way to support your partner and future child. You have the right to be involved and to be kept informed about her care and treatment. Don't let hospital personnel and routines shut you out. Ask questions. Voice your concerns. Stay with her if possible. Some hospitals have policies that exclude the partner from being with the woman during certain exams and procedures. If so, politely question the reasons for your exclusion. If appropriate, convince the hospital staff that she will be better off for your presence and support. She may rely on you to be the more assertive one. The various treatments are preoccupying her now; medications may make her too uncomfortable or too sleepy to assert herself. You may occasionally be left to interact with the health personnel on her behalf. Take the responsibility of staying informed about her condition so you can clarify it to her.

If you can't be present during the doctor's rounds, and you still have questions, find out if the doctor is open to your phone calls. Many physicians encourage using this additional channel of communication as a means of staying in touch with you. You, her partner, play an integral role in her hospital care and can be an invaluable source of support. Providing small comfort measures, talking with the health professionals, and just being there are a greater contribution than you may realize.

Unfortunately, all of your encounters and experiences within the hospital may not go as smoothly as outlined in this chapter. Not every member of the health team has the knowledge or inclination to provide you with explanations and support. You and your partner may need to assert yourselves at times to get the care and information you want. If you are polite and knowledgeable while asserting yourself, you are more likely to get positive results.

You will find that most hospital personnel are courteous and competent, trying to make your stay a pleasant one. However, if you and your partner believe that you are not getting the optimal care you deserve, do speak up. Try to discuss the problem directly with the individual. If that isn't possible or doesn't work, ask to speak with that person's supervisor. Speak with the charge nurse; they are aware of how the various departments and individuals interact and function. Perhaps there is just a personality conflict. If that is the case, ask that a different nurse be assigned to you. If, however, you find one or more nurses you really like, let them know how much you appreciate their expertise. Ask if they can be your nurse on a regular basis. While it is important and sometimes necessary to assert yourself and your needs, remember to do so tactfully and pleasantly so as not to alienate anyone.

Do feel free to ask questions and keep asking questions as time goes on. You have a right and a responsibility to stay informed and to clearly understand your situation. Never feel that your questions or concerns are silly or trivial. Don't let anyone else make you feel that way, either. It is a challenge and a continual effort to stay on top of your circumstances. Some couples feel they don't even know the right questions to ask. Anxiety can easily interfere with rational thinking. If this is your situation, express these feelings to your clinician or a nurse with whom you have a good rapport. They can ease your frustration by providing basic information and reassurance.

7

PRETERM DELIVERY AND THE PREMATURE BABY

My wife was thirty-five weeks pregnant and had been on bedrest for two months, along with oral medications. When she arrived that day at Labor and Delivery, she was bleeding heavily from the vagina from her placenta previa, and therefore an immediate Cesarean section was done. We thought that our son, after so many weeks of being kept inside the uterus, by bedrest and medication, would be ready for the outside world. However, his lungs weren't ready and he was transferred to a nearby university hospital and spent 3 days on a respirator. I remember when my wife and I went for a prenatal visit at thirty weeks, and our obstetrician was telling us how important it was, despite the stress of bedrest, to keep our baby in the womb rather than have a two-lb. infant in the Intensive Care Nursery. That comment didn't mean anything to me until I went to see my son for the first time. The impact of all of those tiny babies all covered with wires and catheters hooked up to big machines was so frightening to me. I was so glad my thirty-five-week-old son was one of the biggest babies there. He was home with us in two weeks.

Jonathan Brown,
father of Jacob (two years).

When early labor leads to preterm birth, the pregnant woman and her partner are usually unprepared. Not only are they often caught without having completed a childbirth preparation course, but they are not acquainted with any of the concepts or terminology of a preterm delivery. After the delivery of a premature baby, the couple usually faces an unfamiliar world in the Newborn Intensive Unit. This chapter is included so that if you do experience a preterm delivery, you will be more knowledgeable about what is happening, and better able to participate actively in the health care of your premature newborn.

THE PRETERM DELIVERY

When a preterm delivery is imminent, the pregnant woman and her partner usually have not completed a childbirth preparation class and are very anxious about not being able to "handle" the labor well. However, the labor of a premature baby is often rapid, and the nurses in the Labor and Delivery Unit are skilled at giving "crash courses" in breathing techniques to parents who might not be totally prepared.

As in all labors, but especially in those of premature babies, it is important that you not take any pain medication unless absolutely necessary. A narcotic that might be routinely used to relieve labor pains in the delivery of a full-term baby (e.g., Demerol, Nisentil) may affect a premature baby profoundly by delaying spontaneous breathing at birth and by complicating the initial assessment of the baby by the pediatrician (in terms of distinguishing the effects of the medication from those of prematurity). However, some experts do suggest that the mother laboring with a premature infant have epidural anesthesia. (See Appendix B for a full explanation of anesthesia.)

Epidural anesthesia during the labor of a premature baby decreases the "urge to push" felt by the laboring mother in the pushing stage. The head of the premature baby is quite soft, and the blood vessels within the brain are more fragile than those of a full-term baby. A tumultuous journey through the birth canal from uncontrollable pushing by the mother may predispose the premature baby to an intracranial hemorrhage (bleeding into the brain), and long term brain damage may result. An epidural anesthetic will decrease this urge to push. If an epidural is used, it is usually placed when the cervix is five cm dilated, as progress from five to ten cm dilated with a small baby is quite rapid, and the epidural needs to be working before the urge to bear down is felt.

Out of consideration for the "soft" head of a premature baby, a generous episiotomy (incision in the vagina) is usually made at birth to protect the head of the baby from any pressure of the vaginal tissues (although a three-pound baby would not usually require an episiotomy for delivery). Some obstetricians routinely use "premature baby forceps" (spoon-like instruments that fit snugly around the head of the baby) to help guide the head of the baby out of the vagina. Other obstetricians prefer to use their hands to cushion the soft head of the premature baby from the pressures of the vaginal tissues.

There is some controversy over whether or not to perform routine Cesarean sections for the births of very small premature infants, as a Cesarean section may be the most gentle of all births. As of this writing, there is no conclusive evidence that premature babies in a "head down" position who are born by Cesarean section have any fewer complications than those born vaginally. Certainly, the mother who undergoes a Cesarean section is subject to the risks of surgery (infection, injury to the bladder, bleeding). However, if a premature baby is in a breech position, the consensus among most obstetricians is that the best mode of delivery is by Cesarean section.

A fetal monitor is used routinely during the labor of a premature baby, as these babies are at increased risk for experiencing fetal distress. Each time the uterus contracts, the blood flow is shut off between the baby and the placenta. For babies at full term with normal placentas, these contractions are usually tolerated well without any dips in the heart rate of the baby, indicating that the baby is not being stressed. However, for premature babies, the placenta may have been compromised (e.g., by placental abruption, causing the preterm labor), and therefore there may be more dips in the fetal heart rate during the stresses of the uterine contractions. This stress is manifested by a pattern of decreased heartbeats in relationship to the contractions. If fetal distress in a premature baby is suspected, occasionally a fetal scalp sample is obtained. This is an evaluation of the acid-based balance of the baby's blood, which reflects directly how much oxygen the baby is receiving. This test is done by obtaining a blood sample from the scalp of the fetus during labor. It is similar to a "finger stick" to check a blood count in the adult. If the heart rate tracing on the monitor, or the fetal scalp sample, indicate that the fetus is in jeopardy, a Cesarean section is performed.

Optimally, the delivery of the premature baby takes place in the delivery room, typically amidst numerous nurses and doctors (usually including an anesthesiologist), all of whom are making preparations to respond to any special needs of the premature newborn. It is very important, despite the chaotic appearance of the delivery room, that the mother and her partner be as relaxed as possible, using slow breathing techniques to ease the arrival of their newborn child gently into the world. (See Chapter Eight on slow breathing techniques.)

Once born, the baby is immediately evaluated by the pediatrician. If initially stable, often the baby can be wrapped in warm blankets and held by the parents for a brief time. However, it is important that the baby be transferred soon to the nursery, for a more thorough evaluation and to be kept warm, as premature newborns get cold very quickly. Therefore, the parents should not expect to have more than a few moments for the initial contact with their baby. If the baby is not doing well at birth, the neonatal team may disappear immediately with the baby. Be assured that as soon as the baby is stabilized, one of the team members will return to inform the parents of the situation. As soon as the baby is stable, one or both parents will be able to go to the nursery to continue the bonding process.

If the baby is transferred from the original hospital where the birth took place to a Level II or III Intensive Care Nursery, the family is often unexpectedly separated. The separation can be quite difficult for all family members, including the partner, who is torn between wanting to be with the newborn and with the mother. The separation can be made easier by transferring the mother to the same hospital as the baby (if she anticipates a lengthy hospital stay), Polaroid pictures of the baby, frequent phone calls to the nurses caring for the baby by family members, and an early discharge of the mother from the original hospital, if medically advisable.

THE PREMATURE BABY

An incredible amount of progress has been made in the medical care of the premature infant in the last twenty years, with the advent of the Neonatal Intensive Care Unit (NICU). What would have been "news" twenty years ago, e.g., the survival of a three-pound infant, is now often taken for granted with the multifaceted support of the NICU. However, the problems involved in the care of a premature infant can be very complex, and the ability of the available technology to help this very tiny newborn can be limited. In order to help you gain an understanding of these problems, we will discuss the development of the fetus in utero, and continue with a description of the problems that premature infants face at various gestational ages.

DEVELOPMENT OF THE FETUS

The miracle of life begins when the egg and sperm meet at ovulation. If a woman has a regular menstrual cycle every twenty-eight days, ovulation occurs around day fourteen. For forty-eight hours following ovulation, the egg can be fertilized by available sperm. If a woman has irregular menstrual cycles, her time of ovulation is most reliably counted two weeks from the first day of her last period. Therefore, if a woman has thirty-five-to thirty-seven-day cycles, she is likely to ovulate between days twenty-one to twenty-three. If you have any doubt regarding your probable time of conception, it is very important that you inform your clinician of this, especially in the situation of premature labor, in which the calculation of the due date is critical. If you had been keeping a basal body temperature chart during the time of conception, be sure to share this chart with your clinician.

Obstetrical language regarding the due date can be confusing. When you are informed that you are eight weeks pregnant, your clinician means that you are eight weeks from the first day of your last menstrual period. However, the baby is really only six weeks old, as the baby exists only from the time of conception. Ideally, the length of pregnancy should be counted from the date of conception. However, tradition states that you use the first day of the last menses as the counting point. In books with pictures of fetuses, when a fetus is described as ten weeks old, that usually means ten weeks old from the first day of the last period. The other confusing aspect of the pregnancy countdown is that pregnancy is described as being nine months long. However, these are lunar months, not four-week months. A normal pregnancy is forty weeks long from the first day of the last menstrual period, which is actually ten four-week months.

Only approximately 4 percent of babies actually deliver on their due dates, with most of them arriving within two weeks before or after the due date. Usually, the babies of women who have been treated successfully for premature labor or weakened cervix arrive between thirty-eight and forty weeks. However, there have been occasional instances of babies going "over" the due date even if a woman has been treated for these conditions. It is important to remember that as the uterus becomes larger during the pregnancy, the uterine muscle becomes more resistant to contractions that earlier could easily efface and dilate the cervix. Therefore, three hours of contractions at twenty-six weeks often signifies imminent delivery, whereas three hours of the same contractions at thirty-seven weeks usually alters the cervix very little.

The fetus forms completely in the first twelve weeks of the pregnancy (counting from the first day of the last menstrual period). Once the egg is fertilized by the sperm, the cells begin to divide. As they divide, they drift down the Fallopian tube into the uterus, where they implant about four days after the time of fertilization. This cluster of cells finds nourishment in the lining of the uterus, and about two weeks from ovulation the embryo begins to form. An ovarian cyst (corpus luteum), which forms at the time of ovulation, now begins to secrete increased amounts of hormone (progesterone) to support the nourishment of the embryo. The placenta (the "afterbirth"), which is attached to the lining of the uterus and is linked to the embryo by an umbilical cord, then begins to form and function. One of the functions of the placenta is to produce HCG (human chorionic gonadotropin), the hormone which is responsible for the increased fatigue in the mother in the first three months, and also for the frequent nausea during the first trimester. The placenta, once formed, also begins to produce progesterone, and thus takes over the function of the corpus luteal cyst of the ovary.

Every vital organ of the embryo is formed in the first two months of life. That is why it is so important during those first two months to avoid medication, radiation exposure, alcohol, etc. At the end of the first month, the embryo is the size of a small pea. By the end of the second month, it is about one inch long. At this point the embryo can move arms and legs, open and close the mouth, and swallow. At the end of the two months, the embryo officially becomes a fetus.

During the third month, the body length of the fetus doubles. The eyelids come together (fuse) and remain closed until the twenty-fifth week of pregnancy. Fingernails appear, and external genital organs are now fully differentiated as either male or female. Often during the third month the heartbeat of the fetus can be detected by a Doppler amplifier in the office, so that you can hear your baby's heartbeat.

During the fourth month, the fetus is often seen sucking a thumb. Very soft "lanugo" hair covers the skin of the fetus. Vernix caseosa forms to protect the skin from the drying effects of amniotic fluid that surrounds the fetus. The amniotic fluid is formed by the secretions of the fetus. This is the fluid that is sampled during an amniocentesis for genetic studies, which is often done in the fourth month of pregnancy.

In the fifth month the fetus grows quite rapidly. Usually the mother is feeling movement at this point in her pregnancy (often at first as "gas pains" or "fluttering"). At this time, the fetus can detect sound and is quite active. During the last four months of pregnancy, the fetus grows from one and a half pounds to seven or eight pounds, and the lungs mature, along with the other vital organs. Below is a chart describing the average weight of the fetus at each gestational week, so that you can measure your progress in terms of your baby's weight at different times.

AVERAGE FETAL WEIGHTS AT
DIFFERENT GESTATIONAL AGES

WEEKS OF GESTATION	WEIGHT IN POUNDS
17	.20
18	.30
19	.40
20	.50
21	.70
22	.80
23	.90
24	1.1
25	1.3
26	1.5
27	1.8
28	2.0
29	2.2
30	2.8
31	3.0
32	3.3
33	3.7
34	4.2
35	4.8

AVERAGE FETAL WEIGHTS AT
DIFFERENT GESTATIONAL AGES

WEEKS OF GESTATION	WEIGHT IN POUNDS
36	5.3
37	5.8
38	6.4
39	6.6
40	7.0

(Adapted from Lubchenco, L. O., by Jeffrey Wasson, M.D., 1985.)

THE PREMATURE INFANT

In general, the survival of the premature infant depends heavily upon the number of weeks of gestation at the time of birth, and the weight of the baby at the time of the birth, independent of the gestational age. No infant has been reported to survive under twenty-two weeks of gestational age. The few infants who have survived between twenty-two and twenty-six weeks of gestational age have guarded long-term prognoses. However, babies who are born after this have increasingly good chances for survival for each week of gestation, although various problems may be encountered along the way. Because these problems are often defined according to the number of weeks of gestation, the discussion will be divided into three parts: borderline prematurity (thirty-seven to thirty-eight weeks gestation), moderate prematurity (thirty-one to thirty-six weeks gestation), and extreme prematurity (fewer than thirty-one weeks gestation).

The Borderline Premature Infant

Infants born at thirty-seven to thirty-eight weeks of gestation usually do very well. Only rarely are the lungs not fully mature at this age. However, if the final lung maturation has not taken place, usually only minimal ventilatory support is needed for an infant at this time (e.g., oxygen over the face under a hood for one to two days). Babies born at this age often do not stabilize their body temperatures well immediately after birth; they become "cold" about five to ten minutes after delivery and may need to be in a "warmer" for a few hours.

Another problem that borderline premature babies may have is jaundice (yellow skin coloring), resulting from an immature liver. Their liver is unable to completely process bilirubin (breakdown products of red blood cells), and the bilirubin remains in the circulation instead of being cleared by the liver, which causes the skin of the newborn to be jaundiced. This jaundice is often noted at about the third or fourth day of life, if it is present. If there is jaundice, a blood test is done. If the level of bilirubin is only mildly elevated, the infant may be given water after feedings and placed near a sunny window (the natural sunlight helps to break up the bilirubin products). If the level of bilirubin is moderately elevated, the infant is placed under the "bili lights." The bilirubin lights are in the blue spectrum of light, and help to break up the potentially dangerous bilirubin products. The lights are usually housed within an incubator. If your baby needs this treatment, a mask is placed over the eyes, to protect them from any deleterious effect of the lights, while the rest of the baby's skin is exposed. It is often necessary to keep the baby under the bili lights for twenty-four to forty-eight hours (the baby is removed from the incubator for feedings).

If the level of bilirubin is dangerously high, an "exchange transfusion" is performed to remove the bilirubin products rapidly from the baby's blood. At this level, possible long-term brain damage can occur, and therefore the exchange transfusion needs to be done promptly. An exchange transfusion consists of removing a portion of the baby's blood with the high concentration of bilirubin products, and replacing it with donor blood to dilute the remaining bilirubin products in the baby's blood. Often, even after the exchange transfusion, the bili lights are needed for several days to help control the bilirubin level.

Infants at thirty-seven to thirty-eight weeks of gestation are occasionally slow to breastfeed or bottlefeed, as they may be easily fatigued. If that happens, your pediatrician may initially recommend supplementing your baby's breastfeeding with formula or water, as it requires much less energy from the baby to suck from a bottle than from the breast, and it is important to keep the baby well hydrated. If your baby is not sucking well at the breast, it is important for you to use the electric breast pump to properly stimulate your milk reflex, so that adequate milk will eventually be produced. Although initially only colostrum will be obtained, the milk will be stimulated to come in, and in a few days one can expect one to two ounces of milk every four hours. It is very important that the mother of a premature baby plan to breastfeed, as the best milk for nourishing the baby is the mother's own breast milk. This breast milk not only provides the essential nutrients appropriate to that age of gestation, but also probably plays a role in preventing colitis (an inflammatory bowel condition), which can develop as a life-threatening complication in a premature newborn infant (see Glossary).

The Moderately Premature Infant

Infants born at thirty-one to thirty-six weeks of gestation have a good chance of survival, although major medical problems are often encountered. These may include respiratory distress syndrome (RDS) or hyaline membrane disease, hypothermia (decreased body temperature), infection, anemia, metabolic imbalance, hypoglycemia (decreased blood sugar); hypocalcemia (low blood calcium), hemorrhage into the central nervous system, colitis of the bowel, and heart problems.

The most common problem of the moderately premature infant is respiratory distress syndrome. From about twenty-four weeks of gestation the lung "buds" exist to support ventilation; however, they do not usually mature until the last four to eight weeks of the pregnancy. If the lungs are not mature in a newborn infant, the baby is often observed to exert a lot of effort in trying to breathe: the baby is breathing rapidly, the nostrils are flaring, and a cyanosis (blue tint) may be seen in the skin coloring. At thirty-five to thirty-six weeks of gestation, about 5 percent of all newborn infants will develop RDS. At thirty-one to thirty-two weeks of gestation, 35 percent of infants will have RDS. Amniocentesis can reliably predict which infant will develop RDS (see Appendix B). If a premature baby is delivered by Cesarean section two to six weeks before the due date, the chance of developing RDS is eight to ten times greater than if a vaginal birth occurs at the same gestational age. (The theory is that the uterine contractions stress the baby and mature the lungs.)

The treatment for RDS can range from simple observation to long-term ventilatory support over many days (e.g., a respirator breathing for the baby). The diagnosis of RDS is made by clinical observation and is confirmed by chest X-ray. Once respiratory distress has been diagnosed, it is important to help the baby breathe, so that the baby is not too fatigued, by providing additional oxygen. The amount of oxygen provided has to be calculated exactly, and may vary from hour to hour. If too much oxygen is given, there may be adverse long-term effects on the baby's vision. Therefore, blood samples are taken at regular intervals for the calculation of the oxygen flow. If the RDS is moderate or severe, an umbilical artery catheter, or "UA line," is usually placed into the umbilical cord of the baby to take direct oxygen measurements. Once the catheter has been placed, an X-ray is taken to confirm that its position is correct (to ensure that the circulation to the legs is not blocked). If the RDS is mild to moderate, sometimes a hard plastic hood with an oxygen flow is placed over the baby's face. If the RDS is severe, a tube is placed into the infant's airway (endotracheal intubation); the tube is attached to a machine (respirator) that provides both the oxygen and the pressure needed to ventilate the baby's lungs. RDS usually worsens over the first twenty-four to seventy-two hours of life, and then gradually improves over the next few days (and sometimes weeks), after which time the respiratory support may no longer be needed.

Occasionally, if the baby needs a respirator for a prolonged period, a condition called bronchopulmonary dysplasia can develop. This condition may represent chronic lung problems that may necessitate prolonged oxygen therapy during the early weeks of life.

Infections can occur in any newborn, but the premature newborn is especially susceptible. These infections can include meningitis (infection of the spinal fluid surrounding the spinal cord and the brain), sepsis (infection of the blood), pneumonia, or a bladder infection. The premature infants especially at risk for the development of these infections are the ones of whom the membranes of the mother have been ruptured before the birth (the longer the membranes have been ruptured, the more risk of infection). Usually, every premature newborn is tested for an infection, even if there has been no previous rupture of the membranes, as any infection can be life-threatening to these tiny infants. Testing for infections usually involves blood tests (CBC, blood cultures), a chest X-ray, a spinal tap (removing a small amount of spinal fluid from the spinal canal via a tiny needle), a urine sample analysis, and an evaluation of the gastric aspirate (a sample of stomach fluid obtained by passing a tube down the mouth of the infant into the stomach). Although it may be difficult for you as a parent to allow your tiny baby to go through such procedures, all of these tests are important. Once the tests are collected, the baby is usually started on antibiotics (e.g., Ampicillin, Gentamacin) for a few days until the test results confirm a lack of infection.

Anemia can also occur in the premature infant. A two-lb. baby may have an anemia caused by the frequent removal of blood for important tests—for instance, oxygen levels. Often premature newborns who have RDS or infections require multiple blood transfusions because of anemia. The average number of blood donors giving blood for transfusions for a single premature baby at the University of California at Los Angeles is nine (different donors).[1] As with any blood transfusion, multiple blood

---

[1] Personal communication with Yvonne Bryson, M.D.

transfusions in a premature baby pose the risk of hepatitis or possibly AIDS (acquired immune deficiency syndrome). In order to minimize the risks of these transfusions, some hospitals have a "walking donor" program in which a NICU nurse, or a family member (once the blood type has been matched), can be the primary donor to the baby needing the blood. This approach may minimize the risk of hepatitis or AIDS to the premature newborn.

Occasionally, a dangerous bowel condition develops in a premature infant: necrotizing enterocolitis (NEC). This condition represents an injury to a part of the intestine, usually resulting from lack of sufficient blood flow to a part of the intestine. If NEC develops, it is usually treated initially with antibiotics and intravenous fluids. In severe cases, surgery to remove the diseased part of the bowel may be necessary. It is thought that a premature baby fed only breast milk has a smaller chance of developing NEC than does a premature baby receiving formula.

Sometimes bleeding can occur within the fragile head of the premature newborn, causing an "intracranial hemorrhage." Intracranial hemorrhages most commonly manifest themselves on the third day of life. The diagnosis is confirmed by an ultrasound of the brain. There are three different levels of intracranial hemorrhage, Level 1 being the least and Level 3 the most severe. Although some babies can recover from a Level 3 intracranial hemorrhage, there may be residual long-term brain damage, e.g., hydrocephalus (see glossary).

Occasionally, a premature baby may develop a heart condition in which a fetal blood vessel connecting two parts of the circulatory system persists and fails to shut down properly once the birth occurs (patent ductus arteriosus). Consequently, some of the blood that is vital to the infant is shunted away from important parts of the body. If the patent ductus arteriosus does not gradually close down over the first few days of life, surgical or drug treatment is necessary to prevent heart failure. The treatment is usually successful and does not present a major obstacle in the recovery of the premature newborn.

Some premature babies stop breathing on their own for short periods of time (apnea spells). If this happens, usually the baby just needs to be stimulated by touching to be reminded to breathe, or occasionally assisted by a puff of oxygen. If apnea spells occur frequently, an apnea monitor is usually attached to the baby to detect these spells. Occasionally, a medication called Aminophylline is administered to premature babies who have repeated apnea spells. Usually the baby simply "outgrows" these spells, if they occur. It is often recommended that parents of a premature newborn being discharged from the nursery take a special CPR (cardiopulmonary resuscitation) course taught by the American Red Cross or by the hospital so that they can take care of any sudden problem that may develop in their babies at home. We recommend this course to all new parents, of both full-term and premature babies.

Hypothermia, or decreased body temperature, is a common problem in premature babies. Body heat is lost very rapidly, so that the babies are often placed under a "radiant warmer" in an open bed, or in an incubator. Once the baby weighs over four pounds, the ability to hold onto their own body heat has usually matured, and the baby can then be transferred to a crib.

Feeding the moderately premature baby is often delayed until the major medical problems are stabilized. During the initial stabilization, fluid intake is usually provided through an intravenous or UA line. These IV fluids contain a balanced salt solution. If long-term IV fluids are needed (e.g., the baby is unable to tolerate feedings because of an immature digestive tract), a hyperalimentation program is begun. Through the IV, fluid that contains all of the essential proteins and calories for growth is administered. Sometimes a premature baby can develop a metabolic acidosis (an acid imbalance), hypoglycemia, or hypocalcemia. In these situations, special supplements are provided through the intravenous line to correct the deficiencies.

Once the medical problems have stabilized, feedings are begun. Often the premature baby will not have the energy required for breastfeeding, and the first feedings are by "gavage" (an infant feeding tube is passed through the mouth into the stomach and a small amount of breast milk or formula is placed through the tube at frequent intervals). Eventually, the baby is able to "nipple" at a bottle or breast.

If at all possible, it is beneficial for your baby to receive your breast milk once feedings are begun. The nurses in the NICU will instruct you in how to maintain your milk supply and how to transport the milk to the NICU. It is important that you start to use the electric breast pump the first day after the birth (these can easily be rented on a weekly basis, and insurance will often cover the cost if your obstetrician writes a letter). Additional information on nursing the premature baby can be found in the Bibliography.

The Extremely Premature Infant

The premature newborn delivered between twenty-five to thirty-one weeks frequently encounters all of the medical problems described above. The amount of time this very tiny newborn spends in the NICU can vary from weeks to months. As parents of this very tiny infant, you have to deal not only with the technology involving your child's care, but also with the worry and the prolonged separation from the baby. Be assured that everything possible is being done, and that often the outcome is excellent.

Overall, the medical problems for a premature infant can be minimal, or they may seem overwhelming. It is important to remember that, in most cases, you will take home a healthy infant. Several long-term follow-up studies have shown that infants who weigh between 3.5 and 5.5 lbs. at birth, and who do not experience RDS, do not differ from children born at term when both groups are evaluated in middle childhood. Among premature infants weighing less than 3.5 lbs. at birth who do survive, about 10 to 20 percent develop handicaps ranging from mild (e.g., hearing loss, learning disability) to major (cerebral palsy, mental retardation). In general, the less complicated the NICU course (i.e., the fewer the problems), the better the long-term prognosis. Often special follow-up pediatric care is recommended for infants born prematurely, so that if problems do develop, early intervention can minimize them.

THE DELIVERY OF MEDICAL CARE
TO THE PREMATURE NEWBORN

It cannot be overemphasized that the optimal facility for the delivery of a premature infant is a hospital that is equipped with a neonatal team appropriate to the degree of prematurity. (See Chapter One for the discussion of Level I, II, and III nurseries.) From the first moment of life, the care of the premature newborn is critical. The neonatal team often consists of a number of people, all of whom will be taking care of the premature baby.

The choice of the primary pediatrician who will care for your baby is a personal one, often based on the philosophy of medical care you may share with that medical practitioner, and proximity to home. While you are on bedrest for preterm labor, it is not too early to choose a pediatrician (or family practitioner, with a pediatrician as backup). One approach to choosing a pediatrician is to ask your obstetrician for a referral to one who is well acquainted with the potential problems of the delivery of a premature baby, and who is also aware of the medications used to treat preterm labor. If you are at home on bedrest and cannot interview prospective pediatricians, talk with them by phone and send your partner to an appointment to meet them. Find out from your obstetrician or pediatrician in which hospital you will deliver, if you do have a premature birth. You might decide to preregister at that hospital, as well as at your own hospital, just to cover all bases.

If you do deliver at a hospital that has a Level I nursery, and problems develop beyond the capacity of that nursery to handle them, the baby will be transferred to a Level II or III NICU. In most NICUs, besides the neonatologist, a variety of resident physicians, fellow physicians, and medical students are involved in the hour-to-hour care of the newborn. (Resident physicians have completed medical school and are in various stages of their training as pediatricians. A neonatology fellow is a pediatrician who is completing a year of specialized training in the care of newborns with problems. Medical students are usually third- or fourth-year students completing their training as physicians.) The members of the neonatal team responsible for the minute-to-minute care of your baby are the NICU nurses. These nurses usually work an eight- to twelve-hour shift. Often one-to-one nursing care is available, so that one nurse will have responsibility for only one baby at a time, and can direct total attention to that one baby.

The physical space of the NICU can be overwhelming: so many tiny babies hooked up to tubes and respirators. Although medical equipment must be present, there are several things that you, as a parent, can do to help your baby know you are there too, and that the world is normally not full of shiny technology. Visit your baby often. Prerecord a tape of your voice so that when you aren't there the nurses can play the tape to the baby. Touch your baby, and help out in any way possible with the care. Put a stuffed animal next to the baby, or hang a colorful mobile nearby. Knit a small cap for your baby. Call in regularly when you can't be there to ask how your baby is doing. Tap all of your resources (your primary care pediatrician, your support group, your childbirth educator) to help facilitate your understanding of what is happening. Usually the NICU team includes a social worker who will also help you get through this stressful period. Often there are organized support groups of parents of premature newborns that can be very valuable during this time. Ask the NICU staff for this information.

The cost of having a baby in a NICU can be staggering, often reaching over $50,000 after a few days. Now is a good time to check your medical insurance policy to be sure your baby will be covered from the first day of life. Some insurance policies do not cover the first thirty days of life, as this is one of the most dangerous times medically for an infant (e.g., if the baby is born prematurely, hospitalization is quite expensive). If you do find that your insurance policy has this rider of not covering the baby for the first thirty days of life, you should investigate other policies.

Obviously, not only is your womb the best medical environment for your unborn baby, but it is also the less expensive alternative, as compared to the cost of the NICU. Therefore, do not be overly concerned with the cost of your hospitalization for premature labor or for your medication; compared to the cost of a potential NICU stay, it is inexpensive.

Every week you gain, as your premature labor is treated, is a week well invested. Knowing the ramifications of a premature birth may help boost your motivation during the taxing days of bedrest during premature labor.

MARSHA'S STORY

It was definitely a high-risk pregnancy. I was forty-two years old and had never before given birth to a child. Within the past three years I had experienced three painful miscarriages, one in the fifth month. I had large fibroid tumors, endometriosis, and severe anemia. Everyone told me that what I needed was a hysterectomy, not another miscarriage.

My husband and I finally had accepted the painful reality that we would not be able to have a child. We adopted a nine-year-old girl and were deeply engaged in adapting to our new role as parents. In May 1982, I discovered that I was pregnant. The due date was February 16, four days before my forty-third birthday. Since we were using birth control, my husband called this pregnancy an accident, but on a deeper level we both knew that we had *chosen* to be careless. Though we had never discussed it, neither of us had really relinquished our desire to have a baby.

The first decision we faced was whether I should go ahead with the pregnancy, since the chances of its succeeding were so dismal (I was already bleeding), and since I now needed to maintain my health to cope with the combined responsibilities of motherhood and of a demanding career. The first year of mothering an adopted older child may not be physically taxing, but it is certainly emotionally turbulent. Since it was my health that was at risk, my husband felt that the decision whether or not to continue the pregnancy should be mine. Most of my friends and loved ones were against it, because they thought I was jeopardizing my health to pursue an unrealistic dream. I decided to go ahead. Since this would definitely be my last pregnancy, I committed myself to doing everything humanly possible to give this child life.

The next decision I had to make was whether to change doctors. For the past five years I had been going to the same group of doctors. Since I had had so many gynecological problems, I had chosen my doctor very carefully. The head doctor in the office had the reputation of being the best gynecologist in the city. I had heard that judgment from a number of sources, including several other doctors. Since he was now nearing retirement age, he was no longer handling pregnancies. The obstetrician who had attended me during my three miscarriages was rather young (at least, younger than I). I found him intelligent, knowledgeable, kind, yet there was something about his practice that made me uneasy. When my miscarriages had occurred, he had consoled me by saying "it was nature's way of taking care of things." Before my first miscarriage, when I had asked him whether he thought bedrest was necessary, since I was experiencing light bleeding, he said that no one really knew whether it did any good and that I could maintain my normal level of activity, but not overdo it. After my water sac broke in the fifth month, I was confined to total bedrest, but one week later the umbilical cord fell out of my body and the baby was born dead. In my next two pregnancies (which ended in the third and second months respectively), I was not told to take any special precautions. His remark about "nature's way of taking care of things" kept ringing in my ears. I realized that he and his colleagues did not have a special strategy for dealing with high-risk pregnancies. Another thing that made me uneasy was that they had just acquired a new ultrasound machine in their office and were learning how to use it. I could see that my doctor was playing with it like a toy. After examining me on this machine one day, he told me that he thought I had had twins and that one of them had died—that was probably why I was bleeding, and why there was a big spot floating in my uterus. When I had a subsequent ultrasound test on more specialized equipment, the dead twin turned out to be one of the fibroids that had been present through all four pregnancies, and which he had never recommended removing. I didn't want to be unfair to the doctors and blame them for my own physical limitations; yet I knew that if this final pregnancy were going to break the pattern and succeed, I would have to take a different course of action.

A friend told me about another obstetric group, three doctors who specialized in high-risk pregnancies. I made an appointment for an examination and consultation with one of the practitioners, who described their approach to cases like mine. I liked what I heard. Their approach seemed much more active; there was no talk of nature taking its course, but of new drugs and surgical procedures that helped to delay the onset of premature labor. Yet the group's offices were much further from my home, and they were affiliated with hospitals also at a greater distance. I remembered those desperate rides to the hospital for emergency treatment, rides that had seemed endless. Also, these new doctors weren't familiar with my long, complex gynecological history. But this familiarity hadn't enabled my own doctors to prevent miscarriages in the past. I agonized over the decision for a week or so, read whatever I could find about high-risk pregnancies, and finally chose to change doctors. Once the decision was made I felt much more confident and optimistic. I informed my former doctor, and he wrote me a kind letter wishing me luck.

Because of my past history of miscarriages and the fact that I was still bleeding, my new doctors strongly recommended that I remain on bedrest during the entire pregnancy. This put a heavy burden on my husband and daughter, who had to do all the household tasks that I normally did. Being a college professor, I had the summer free, but in September I was scheduled to teach two classes. I was very fortunate, for everyone at the university was very cooperative. I was allowed to drop one class without financial penalty and teach the other, a graduate seminar, in my home. The students came to my house once a week for lectures and discussion and seemed to enjoy the informal atmosphere; my teaching assistant brought me everything I needed from campus. In this way, I avoided going on disability; but even more important, this scaled-down activity provided the intellectual stimulation that made several months of bedrest bearable.

In the fourth month I was scheduled to have amniocentesis. Because of the size of my fibroid tumors, which grew rapidly during the pregnancy, and the low volume of amniotic fluid, the test had to be delayed a few more weeks. Finally we learned that the baby's genes were fine, and that he was a boy. My husband and I immediately began to argue about what to name him.

Despite my remaining on bedrest and following the doctor's orders very precisely, my cervix still began to dilate, which meant I was in danger of going into premature labor. Fortunately I was seeing the doctors quite frequently and they detected the change very early, immediately hospitalizing me so that they could perform a cerclage, a surgical procedure in which the cervix is sutured to prevent dilation. I also began taking Ritodrine, a drug that treated the premature contractions that I was having. The surgery was very successful, the baby's heartbeat continued to be very strong, and we were soon allowed to return home to our bedrest.

Though by now I knew that this was the most difficult pregnancy I had ever experienced, I felt relatively at ease, for I knew that everything humanly possible was being done to give this baby a chance to live. My doctor kept telling me that she had a good feeling about this baby; her instincts told her that he would make it. So did mine.

On Thanksgiving I was feeling particularly strong. I decided to help cook the turkey, which was a mistake. A couple of friends were joining us for dinner, people I knew would be willing to help serve and clean up. Though I spent most of the day in bed, I overexerted myself and overate. But I told myself nothing could go wrong on Thanksgiving—it would be too unfair, too ironic, too corny. Late that night I was physically uncomfortable and couldn't fall asleep. I had stomach pains, gas pains I thought, but by early morning suspected I might be going into labor. I called the doctor's exchange and reached one of the practitioners. I was told to take more Ritodrine and come to the hospital immediately for an examination. By the time I got there, my doctor told me I was definitely in labor and tried various intravenous drugs to arrest the process, since the oral medications had not been successful.

Around midday on Friday, I went to the hospital's ultrasound lab to determine how the baby was doing. In the middle of the examination, my water sac broke. The technician didn't realize what had happened and told me to calm down, but I insisted he go and get the doctor immediately. For the first time, I felt I was going to lose the baby and that nightmare of my first miscarriage was recurring.

There was no going back, the baby was going to be born in the twenty-eighth week of gestation. I was immediately transferred by ambulance to a research hospital with one of the best neonatal intensive care units in the city. My baby's chances for survival were not good, but they would be better there. The sad irony was that the delivery would be performed, not by a practitioner from the group whom I had chosen so carefully and had come to admire, but by the unknown hospital staff.

At the university hospital, I kept meeting new doctors, medical students, and nurses, and could hardly tell one from another. I sorely missed having one of my own doctors, with whom I had established such a strong personal connection. But my husband was with me. They told us they would try to delay the birth as long as possible in order to strengthen the baby's lungs, but that if they left him in too long without the amniotic fluid that had been lost, he risked a bad infection. Since it was late Friday night, they told my husband to get some sleep, and that they would call him as soon as something happened. He went to a friend's house near the hospital. The nurse took his number and promised to call.

After a couple of hours, when the labor pains grew more frequent and intense, I was rushed into the delivery room to have the suture removed from my cervix. Because this was done during the labor pains, it was an agonizing experience. When I was wheeled back into the labor room, I asked the nurse to please call my husband, and she said she would. The labor pains were coming very fast, and I kept calling for the doctor, now remembering a terrible fact about my first miscarriage that I had completely repressed: at that time, despite all of the impressive computerized monitors at the hospital, at the precise moment that my baby boy was expelled from my body, I had been lying in the labor room alone. Later they would tell me he had been born dead.

Now, the nurse finally came and I told her I could feel the baby coming. She didn't believe me and turned to check the monitor. I insisted she get the doctor, any doctor, and I reminded her again to call my husband. The doctors came a few minutes later, and then had to run my stretcher back to the delivery room. We just made it, just barely. It was 7:15 on Saturday morning, November 27. After one more labor pain the baby slipped out and was immediately surrounded by five doctors. All I could see were doctors' backs. I asked, "Is he dead?" Then I heard a brief cry, and they rushed him out of the room. I didn't even get a glimpse. I felt deeply depressed and drained, robbed of all the joy I had expected to come with this birth. I doubted he would live.

The afterbirth came without difficulty. Then a doctor wanted to examine me to see if there was any damage. I told him it was painful. Another doctor told him to wait—they could give me a pain shot now, since the baby was out and I had had no anesthetic. But the first doctor refused to wait the few minutes for the drug to take effect. I felt angry and told him so, but he went ahead anyway. I felt very helpless.

A third doctor, apparently the one in charge, told me that they were now going to give me a general anesthetic so that they could do a more thorough examination. I couldn't believe it. I had gone through this painful experience without any anesthetic and now, in this weakened, depressed condition, they were going to give me a general! What the hell for? He claimed they wanted to see what had caused the premature labor. I told him I knew—it was the fibroids. And since there was no way they were going to take them out now, why should I be subjected to this probing? He told me to be reasonable. If I ever wanted to have another child, this information would be essential. I told him I was forty-two years old and knew for a fact that I would never get pregnant again, and thus had no use for this information. I absolutely refused to have a general anesthetic. He conceded that I had the right to refuse, but told me I was preventing them from learning something valuable. And then I realized that they wanted this information for *their* research, not because it would benefit *me*. I felt very good about resisting the pressure of these doctors, even in my weakened condition, and this thought made me feel stronger.

My husband didn't get to the hospital until I had been in the recovery room for over an hour. No one from the hospital had called him. When I got to my own room, I could already walk to the bathroom. My husband went to check on our baby and found he was still alive, but we didn't know in what condition.

Later that day we went to the Neonatal Intensive Care Unit and saw him for the first time. It was a terrifying room—full of bright lights and massive machines with alarm signals screeching every few minutes. Our two-and-a-half-pound baby was lying on his back in an incubator, with a breathing tube down his throat, an IV in his arm, another line in the heel of his foot, his eyes masked to protect him from the bright lights overhead. We could see our baby's scrawny arms and spidery hands feebly struggling to tear away all the wires and tubes that ensnared him; I had the same impulse. The next time we saw him, his arms were bound at his sides.

Gradually we got used to that room, appreciating that we could come visit our boy at any hour day or night, appreciating the excellent round-the-clock care of the nurses and doctors. Eventually we got to hold him, with all of his wires still attached, but soon they began to disappear. We came twice a day to deliver the breast milk that I was frantically pumping at home, to hold him, or just to be there.

We were very fortunate. His heart and lungs were strong. He was off the respirator in a couple of days. He developed no side effects or complications. After two months in the Neonatal Intensive Care Unit, we brought him home.

Today he is a healthy, vibrant, mischievous two-year-old toddler. We call him Victor.

Marsha Kinder Bautista,
mother of Victor (two years)
and Gabriela (twelve years).

CHILDBIRTH PREPARATION AND PREMATURE LABOR

by Mary Sue Ulven, R.N.[1]

> *Childbirth classes? For someone with premature labor? I
> was thinking of taking them later, but now I may deliver
> before I finish them! Are they still worthwhile?*

Pregnancy is always a time of numerous changes and stresses that involve
the entire family. If you are prospective parents who must also cope with
the stresses of preterm labor, you face an even more difficult challenge. It
is important that expectant couples, especially couples with high-risk pregnancies, find resources that will help them—resources offering practical
information, coping tools, and emotional support. Childbirth preparation
classes are uniquely designed to meet many of the special needs of any
expectant couple.

WHAT DO CHILDBIRTH CLASSES OFFER?

Childbirth classes are attended by the pregnant woman and her support
person. Usually this support person, called the "labor coach," is her partner, although it may be anyone who is close to the woman and intends to
be at the birth. Generally, the focus of any childbirth preparation program

---

[1] Mary Sue Ulven, R.N., is a labor and delivery nurse at Santa Monica Hospital
(Santa Monica, California), and a certified childbirth educator (A.S.P.O.).

is threefold: education, relaxation-based coping skills, and emotional support. There is an abundance of misinformation and superstitions surrounding pregnancy and birth. Consequently, many prospective parents face labor and delivery with great apprehension and fear. Childbirth classes help dispel these fears and misconceptions through education and factual information.

A basic understanding of pregnancy, labor, birth, and the postpartum period provides a sense of preparedness. A wide variety of topics related to pregnancy and childbirth are discussed in the classes, from anatomy and physiology of pregnancy, through stages of labor, to hospital procedures and complications. Emphasis is placed on understanding the process as a way of coping. You are encouraged to ask questions and participate. Possible options and alternatives in birth procedures are discussed, as is how to communicate openly with your obstetrical practitioner and hospital personnel. Knowledge about pregnancy and birth allows you and your partner to participate actively in your health care. This ability to be involved in the decision making provides a greater sense of control over what is happening. Those prospective parents who perceive themselves as having control during pregnancy and the birth subsequently are much more pleased and satisfied with their individual birth experiences.[2]

The second focus of childbirth preparation classes is conscious relaxation. Relaxation training is one of the most valuable ways to prepare not only for childbirth, but for any stressful or anxiety-producing situation. Genuine relaxation requires consciously recognizing and releasing tension in the body. Tension is often habitual, misdirecting the body's energy into headaches, backaches, muscle stiffness, insomnia, and a variety of other tension-related physiological and psychological responses. The stresses of pregnancy often increase these symptoms of tension. Practiced regularly, conscious relaxation interrupts this cycle of stress and tension, revitalizing the body and the mind.[3] When the body is not wasting energy in tension, there is less fatigue. The body then works more efficiently, as tense muscles are no longer taking oxygen that could be better used by the uterus and the baby. Relaxation also gives you an increased awareness of your own body, providing intuitions about how best to help yourself and, again, increasing your sense of control. Because relaxation techniques reduce perception of pain and increase pain tolerance, they are the basis for the breathing techniques taught to cope with the discomforts of labor. Such

---

2. Willmuth, L. Prepared childbirth and the concept of control. *JOGN Nursing,* 4(5):38–41, 1975.

3. Benson, H. *The Relaxation Response.* New York: Avon Books, 1976.

techniques require a controlled mind and a relaxed body for maximum benefit.

The third focus of childbirth education classes is emotional support. The emotional well-being of the expectant woman affects not only her ability to cope, but also her physical health and that of her baby. Numerous studies have shown that a high anxiety level may predispose the woman to increased complications of pregnancy.[4] The woman in labor with a supportive person in attendance who is emotionally meaningful to her, tends not only to cope better with the labor process but also to have fewer medical complications.[5]

Childbirth classes provide the labor coach with specific techniques and skills that can be used to support the expectant mother and increase her comfort. Communication is also emphasized, and communication skills enhanced. Both partners need support from each other at this time. Sharing the birth of a child means working hard together to cope with the many changes. No matter how good your relationship, conflicts cannot be avoided; the added stresses and new issues surrounding the prospective birth must be worked out. Communication often breaks down when partners don't want to burden each other or think that their concerns are silly. Keeping communication open by sharing anxieties, fears, and concerns is a valuable way of supporting each other, and will strengthen your relationship. Preparing together for the birth is also a valuable first step in preparing to be a good parent team.

The class itself often becomes a source of support to the prospective parents involved. Interacting with other pregnant couples provides reassurance, information, mutual problem solving, and camaraderie. Class members become closer as they share due dates and common experiences of pregnancy. Discussing the shared concerns of expectant parents is also a valuable means of reducing anxiety and increasing coping abilities.

[4.] Zax, M., Sameroff, A., and Farnum, J. Childbirth education, maternal attitudes, and delivery. *Am J Obstet Gynecol,* 123:185–190, 1975.

[5.] Sosa, R., Kennell, J., Klaus, M., Robertson, S., and Urrutia, J. The effect of a supportive companion on perinatal problems, length of labor, and mother-infant interaction. *N Engl J Med,* 303:597, 1980.

CHILDBIRTH EDUCATION
AND THE PREMATURE
LABOR EXPERIENCE

Expectant parents who are experiencing preterm labor have all the concerns of any expectant couple, plus several more. The very real prospect of delivering early may leave you feeling unprepared for the birth experience, unready to be parents, and overwhelmed by all the implications of a preterm birth. Although the possibility of preterm delivery is real, the probability has been greatly reduced in recent years as medical knowledge about preterm labor has increased. However, the methods of treatment for the woman in preterm labor often further impede preparing for the birth. Complete bedrest limits many of the preparations prospective parents enjoy—shopping for the baby, preparing the nursery, baby showers, and socializing. Attending childbirth preparation classes often becomes more important when you are struggling with the increased stresses of a high-risk pregnancy. The classes frequently become the highlight of a week filled with boredom for the woman and with extra work for her partner. They provide much needed information, coping tools, and support, making the baby and prospective birth more real—reinforcing the knowledge that this trying period will eventually end.

You also have a greater need for the information offered in childbirth classes. The woman must often undergo extra medical tests and procedures; you both have added concerns about her health and about the baby. Knowledge about the woman's body and the normal changes of pregnancy provides a basis for understanding the complications as well. Most childbirth instructors include some information about high-risk pregnancy in their classes, and can often suggest other valuable resources. Such knowledge makes it easier for you to understand and accept your situation; then you can discuss it more openly and knowledgeably with your obstetrical practitioner.

Any high-risk situation creates more stress and the need for additional support systems. Preterm labor often turns pregnancy into a long, tedious, anxiety-ridden confinement. Sources of support are harder to find and maintain as friends and relatives go on with their busy lives. Childbirth classes provide contact with other couples who may be in a similar situation. All expectant parents experience pregnancy-related frustrations; the group can be a valuable outlet for emotions that nonpregnant friends and family may not understand.

There are only a few minor restrictions the couple with preterm labor needs to observe in childbirth classes. Since bedrest is an important part of your treatment, you will need to lie down throughout the class. Take a bedroll or sleeping bag and pillows with you so you will be comfortable. You need not feel self-conscious about lying down when everybody else is sitting. Explain your situation, and the other couples will certainly understand; soon no one will think twice about the fact that you're always lying down.

If exercises are taught in class, check with your obstetrical practitioner about which ones are appropriate or inappropriate for you. In general, abdominal exercises are inadvisable. However, stretching exercises done lying down and the pelvic tilt are usually allowed, and may provide relief from the discomforts of bedrest. However, if any of the exercises stimulates uterine contractions, do not do them. When the instructor teaches pushing, listen to the information but definitely do not actually push or bear down. The straining can increase the pressure of the baby on the cervix, and may stimulate contractions. Simply pretend you are pushing, while assuming the positions.

In recent years, many hospitals have relaxed their restrictions regarding who can be with a woman in labor. Check with the hospital where you intend to deliver. If someone in addition to your partner will be allowed in with you, consider recruiting a second labor coach. First labors are often long. Many couples preparing for birth realize the advantages of having two support persons for the laboring woman. This is an excellent idea for the couple who has been through the rigors of preterm labor. The two coaches can provide maximal coaching, support each other as well as the woman, and relieve each other for breaks. If you like this idea, discuss with your partner who among your friends and relatives might be appropriate. Who is sensitive, supportive, and wants to attend the birth? Your baby's birth is a special occasion, so pick a special person. Choose someone who is close to both you and your partner; someone who will be involved but won't take over. Although not absolutely necessary, the backup coach may want to attend a few of your childbirth classes. Ask your instructor if this is possible. Most important, the three of you need to discuss ahead of time the role of the coaches and what your individual needs and goals are for the birth.

RELAXATION AND "THE BREATHING"

The various relaxation and breathing techniques taught in childbirth classes are of more immediate value to the couple with preterm labor. Relaxation and visualization exercises (discussed in more detail in Chapters Two and Ten) not only relieve anxiety and tension, but may also decrease the preterm labor contractions. The woman on bedrest has ample time to practice regularly the various relaxation techniques and discover what works best for her. Busy partners who make time for these exercises will also benefit. Doing the techniques together is a nice way to relax together and harmonize the different energy levels of the two of you.

Many people think of "the breathing" as the main focus of childbirth classes. Actually, the relaxation exercises provide the foundation for learning the specific breathing techniques. Taught for use in coping with the discomforts of labor contractions, these techniques can be applied in any situation that involves physical or mental discomfort. As the woman in preterm labor is often subjected to a greater number of various uncomfortable examinations and procedures, these techniques are of value long before the onset of true labor.

"Slow-Paced Breathing"[6]

The breathing techniques taught in childbirth preparation classes aim to promote relaxation, decrease perception of discomfort, and enhance optimal use of the body's energy. The basic technique is an easily learned, slow, even breathing pattern combined with attention focusing:

1. To begin, count your respirations for one minute (breath in/breath out equals one respiration).

2. Now position yourself comfortably and do a relaxation exercise from Chapter Two (pp. 62–64).

3. After the relaxation exercise, note the pattern of your breathing. You will probably find that your respirations are slow, smooth, and rhythmical, with your chest and abdomen slowly rising and falling. Again count your respirations for one minute. If you succeeded in relaxing your body and mind even slightly, you will find your breaths are slower, deeper, and more rhythmic. When you consciously breathe in this manner, you are doing the slow-paced breathing!

When your body and mind relax, your breathing naturally changes to this slow, restful pattern. Conversely, when you consciously alter your breathing to this pattern, your body and mind will relax. Breathing pat-

---

6. Hilbers, S. Paced Breathing: Terminology changes and teaching techniques. *Genesis*, 5(6):16–18, 1983–84.

terns can influence and also be influenced by your thoughts and emotions. When you alter your breathing pattern voluntarily, you can change both your subjective and physiological experiences.

Practice is necessary to learn to respond to discomfort or anxiety with a slower breathing pattern instead of with fear and tension. Two or three times a day, take five to ten minutes to practice this slow-paced breathing:

1. Settle yourself in a comfortable position with your head, arms, and legs well supported.

2. Clear your mind with a breath that may be a little deeper and longer than usual, a "cleansing breath."

3. Focus your attention on your breathing as you smoothly and evenly inhale and exhale. Feel the air entering your lungs as you inhale, and feel your body going looser with each exhalation. Keep breathing in and out as your chest and abdomen slowly rise and fall in a harmonious, effortless manner.

4. Keep your face, mouth, and tongue relaxed.

5. Never hold your breath! Maintain an easy, smooth flow without pausing at the peak of inspiration.

6. Keep your attention on your breathing pattern. If your mind wanders, gently bring it back to focus on your breath.

The frequency of this slow-paced breathing technique then is approximately half your normal rate (about six to ten breaths per minute). Find your individual rhythm and rate that enables you to obtain maximum calmness and relaxation. How you inhale and exhale is also individual: you can inhale and exhale through your nose; inhale and exhale through your mouth; or inhale through your nose and exhale through your mouth. Nose breathing usually feels the most natural, but experiment for yourself. Many pregnant women experience nasal congestion, and thus find mouth breathing easier. There is great individual variation in the relaxation response; you must find for yourself what best helps you to stay relaxed.

Focusing your attention is an additional tactic to augment the effect of the breathing pattern. Don't let your mind wander; it will most likely wander to thoughts or sensations that interrupt the relaxation process. Focusing calms your mind and puts discomfort in the background of your awareness. There are many strategies for focusing:

1. Focus on some aspect of your breathing: the steady rhythm; the feel of your lungs expanding and contracting; the sound of your breathing; the feel of the air entering and leaving your nose.

2. Counting can be a focus; count slowly as you inhale, and repeat the same count as you exhale, e.g., "in-two-three-four/ out-two-three-four."

3. Find an external focus: rest your eyes and attention on a picture, or perhaps just a spot on the wall, as you breathe.

4. Repeat positive, rhythmic phrases to yourself as you breathe:
   "Breathe in oxygen—breathe out tension"
   "Breathe for the baby—breathe away the pain"
   "Energy in—negative thoughts out"
   "I am safe—I am sound"[7]

The "Cleansing Breath" is another coping strategy to combine with the slow-paced breathing. Similar to a sigh or a yawn, it is slightly deeper and longer and most commonly used at the beginning and end of a contraction. Slowly inhale through your nose with your mouth closed; feel your lungs expanding. Now slowly exhale through your mouth. Use this cleansing breath as a signal to your body and mind that you are going to relax. Each time you do the slow-paced breathing, take a cleansing breath at the beginning and at the end. If you are using this slow breathing during an uncomfortable procedure and still find yourself getting tense, you may find it helpful to inject a cleansing breath and then return to the slow breathing.

This slow-paced breathing is the basic pattern taught in Lamaze classes and is similar to the slow breathing taught in all other childbirth preparation classes. Other patterns that may be taught for different stages of labor are based on this one. You must practice it, however, and become familiar with it for it to work in stressful or uncomfortable situations. Use the preterm contractions to practice this breathing. Although preterm labor is not usually painful, these contractions give you a good sense of what active labor contractions will be like. The contractions gradually build to a peak tightness and then wane as the uterus relaxes. Whenever you feel a preterm contraction, it is an excellent opportunity to practice your breathing technique. The next time you go to your clinician's office or must undergo an uncomfortable procedure, experiment again with this

---

7. Hilbers, S. Op. cit.

breathing pattern. Incorporate it into your lifestyle. The more you use slow-paced breathing, the better it will serve you.

CHOOSING A CHILDBIRTH PREPARATION CLASS

In many communities, there are a variety of prepared childbirth methods from which to choose. All methods have similar histories and philosophies —to educate, support, and provide coping skills for the expectant couple. They differ in emphasis and in some of the specific techniques. There are many factors to consider when choosing a childbirth preparation class. The couple coping with premature labor has additional needs and must carefully consider the classes available to them.

The first choice must be whether to take private or group classes. Discuss this issue with your obstetrical practitioner. Does your activity level allow you to attend weekly group classes? If your situation requires strict bedrest at all times, private classes in your home may be your only option. Private classes are usually more expensive than group classes and often are condensed into two to four lessons instead of the six to eight lessons offered in group classes. If you are unable to leave your home or have exceptionally high chances of early delivery, private classes are probably your best choice.

If at all possible, try to attend group classes. Explain to your practitioner that these classes are very important to you. Suggest that you might take a bedroll and lie down through the class, observing any restrictions deemed necessary. The advantages of group classes over private classes are many. Just to get out of the house for an evening is often a welcome respite from the confinement accompanying preterm labor. Interacting with other expectant parents is a valuable and enjoyable way to gather information. Learning is often enhanced in a group of people who share a common experience. The questions and discussions of the group are often more educational than a didactic private lesson might be. As couples get to know and identify with each other, the atmosphere of the classes is one of caring, concern, and support. Even if the other couples in the class are not familiar with preterm labor, they still share with you many of the other experiences of pregnancy. This commonality reinforces the healthy aspects of your pregnancy. Preparing for labor and delivery reinforces your awareness that a difficult time will come to an end.

Take some time to investigate the childbirth preparation classes available in your community. Your clinician and the Labor and Delivery Unit of the hospital where you intend to deliver are possible resources for suggestions and referrals to teachers in the area. Feel free to interview several childbirth educators; choose someone with whom you feel a rapport and whose class seems best suited to meet your needs. Consider the following when choosing a childbirth preparation class:

1. Instructor qualifications. Background, training, and teaching experience vary widely among childbirth educators.

What training have they had?

How long have they been teaching?

Are they members in good standing of a recognized professional childbirth organization?

Most important, are they familiar with preterm labor, its treatment and the ramifications?[8]

A childbirth educator who is also an obstetrical nurse will probably be more knowledgeable about preterm labor and more aware of your special concerns.

2. Starting the class. Can you enter a class that starts soon? Most childbirth educators enroll couples in a class that ends two to four weeks before their due dates. Couples coping with preterm labor may need and want to take the classes earlier, often as soon as possible after the diagnosis of premature labor. Although many women with preterm labor do carry their pregnancies to term, the concerns and anxieties about an early delivery persist. Taking early classes provides reassurance that you will have the necessary information and skills to cope with labor and delivery whenever it occurs. If you will finish the class well ahead of your due date, ask if you can attend a refresher class or repeat a particular class later when labor and delivery are more imminent.

3. Class size. How many couples in the class? In general, the smaller the group the better. Twelve couples should be the maximum; six to ten couples is preferable. Smaller classes provide more personal attention and more interaction with other class members.

4. Number of hours of instruction time. Most classes are two to three hours once a week for six to eight weeks. Total class time should be a

---

8. Adapted from "Choosing a Childbirth Preparation Class," ASPO of Los Angeles, Inc. 1982.

minimum of twelve hours. Longer classes may provide additional class content.

5. Class content. Most childbirth preparation classes offer the same basic information, but the depth and emphasis vary widely. The couple in premature labor needs a class that emphasizes relaxation skills and also provides in-depth, unbiased information about all aspects of labor and delivery. Time allotted for group discussions and supervised practice of techniques promotes optimal learning. Ask specific questions about the class content:

> What specific subjects are covered?
>
> Is relaxation training a main focus?
>
> Are various relaxation exercises taught?
>
> What percentage of class time is devoted to lecture? to discussion? to practice of techniques?
>
> Are variations from normal labor discussed? Which ones? (e.g., induction of labor, forceps, Cesarean section)
>
> Are the benefits as well as the risks of various hospital procedures and medical interventions discussed? (e.g., monitoring, medication, anesthesia, episiotomy)
>
> Is the emphasis on you and the health care professionals working together as a team to make the right choices for your individual birth experience?
>
> Is the instructor available for questions either before or after class or by phone?

While preterm labor may complicate your expectations and preparations, the birth of your child remains a special time. Use this time to invest in preparing for parenthood; spend the necessary amount of time to find the right childbirth preparation class for you. Read a wide variety of books to supplement your current knowledge about parenting, breastfeeding, and infant care (see Bibliography). Take every opportunity to prepare yourselves for your unique birth experience.

NUTRITION AND EXERCISE IN
A PREGNANCY COMPLICATED
BY WEAKENED CERVIX
OR PREMATURE LABOR

NUTRITION

In any pregnancy, nutrition is of vital importance. Because you are on bedrest, it may be more difficult for you to continue your good nutritional habits. Your appetite may be diminished as a result of inactivity, you may experience heartburn, and you may be unable to choose favorite foods as before because of practical problems in shopping and preparation. It is very important to choose your sources of nutrition carefully, since maternal weight gain is important to the growth of the fetus. The more the baby weighs at birth, the better the chance of survival, if the baby is born prematurely. However, this weight gain should not come from "foods with empty calories," but from foods from healthy sources providing the much-needed building blocks for the growth of the fetus.

As a general guideline, any pregnant woman should consume approximately eighty grams of protein per day. Four glasses of milk (or the equivalent in milk products) per day provide about thirty-five grams of protein. A serving of tuna fish has about twenty-five grams of protein. Other good sources of protein include chicken, soy products, and nuts. Fresh vegetables and fruit are also very important in your nutrition. Foods that encourage regular bowel movements without straining, e.g., roughage such as salads and whole grains, should be added regularly to the diet, as bedrest may decrease normal bowel activity and predispose you to constipation.

It is important to have good sources of calcium. Four servings of milk products along with the calcium in your prenatal vitamin provide you with adequate calcium. However, if you do not consume milk products, it is important to take a separate calcium supplement, as well as eating other food high in calcium (e.g., salmon, broccoli).

Because patients with premature labor may be at increased risk for a complicated birth (e.g., for Cesarean section) it is essential that an iron supplement (separate from the prenatal vitamin) be taken regularly, along with iron-rich foods (liver, spinach, apricots, etc.). This supplemental iron helps to ensure that if unexpected bleeding occurs at the time of the delivery, you have extra iron reserves built up within your body. Having extra iron reserves decreases the possibility that a blood transfusion (with its risks) will be needed.

Certain nutritional restrictions are appropriate for pregnancy, and expecially for the woman on bedrest. It is important to avoid all alcohol intake, although an occasional glass of wine may be prescribed by your clinician if there is an increase in uterine contractions, and the choice is between a glass of wine and a trip into the hospital. It is now known that even moderate drinking (two to three drinks per day) can affect the fetus adversely, not only in the first three months of pregnancy but possibly throughout the remainder of the pregnancy. Pregnant women do have an increased need for salt, which is usually met through a normal diet. However, excessive salt, e.g., routinely adding table salt to food, should be avoided, as this extra salt may encourage the body to hold onto excess fluid, with subsequent swelling of the hands and feet.

Caffeine should be avoided in any pregnancy, but especially in a pregnancy in which there is limited activity and possible medication. Caffeine increases the heart rate. If a woman already has an increased heart rate from taking a medication for the treatment of premature labor, and caffeine might further accelerate the heart rate and cause cardiac symptoms (e.g., chest pain). Foods that contain caffeine include chocolate, dark teas, coffee, and many soft drinks.

For all pregnant women, and especially for women who are on medication to treat premature labor, it is important to decrease sources of concentrated sugar. Intake of fruit or fruit juice should be limited to two to three servings per day. All sugary desserts and cookies should be excluded. The reason is that as soon as a concentrated source of sugar is consumed, the glucose concentration in the mother's blood rises. The subsequent insulin rise in the mother to compensate for the sudden glucose rise often "overshoots," and an hour later the blood of the expectant mother is hypoglycemic (low blood sugar). This rapid shift in glucose range goes directly across to the fetus. The fetus does much better with a constant level of glucose than a rapidly fluctuating level. If you have a sweet tooth, occasional treats can be permitted but should be eaten slowly and in conjunction with some protein. For women on medication to treat premature labor contractions (e.g., Ritodrine), an increased glucose concentration usually occurs as a result of the medication. Therefore, the restraints on sugar intake should be very strict to avoid the development of diabetes in the pregnancy.

EXERCISE

Exercise is important in pregnancy, not only to increase your strength as your baby grows bigger and your weight increases, but also to build up your endurance for an often strenuous labor. Many physiological changes occur in pregnancy. As the uterus grows, cardiovascular changes occur as the fetus needs more and more nutrition and oxygen to flow across the placenta. At about twenty-seven weeks of pregnancy, the volume of blood flow across the placenta is maximal. Often the pregnant woman's heart rate, and occasionally her blood pressure, increase to accommodate this extra blood volume that her heart must deliver across the placenta. Different muscle groups in the body also have to adapt to the changes in the body of a pregnant woman, e.g., back muscles must counterbalance the protruding uterus. It is important to strengthen both the muscles and the cardiovascular system to help your body adapt to these pregnancy changes.

Pregnant women vary in the amount of exercise they need. Currently, there is controversy over how much and which type of exercise a pregnant woman should have on a daily basis. Some exercise is important for the reasons stated above; however, for some women, too much exercise can increase the mother's risk of injury (e.g., the risk of ligament sprain while running increases as a result of laxness of the ligaments caused by pregnancy hormones). Vigorous aerobic exercise may put the fetus in temporary jeopardy (e.g., a maternal heart rate over 120 may deplete the fetus of needed oxygen because in this situation the maternal blood flow is preferentially directed away from the uterus to the mother's brain and kidneys: "survival mode").

In general, exercise during pregnancy should include a variety of exercises for the different parts of the body, and should be done daily. Once an exercise regimen is begun, the amount can be increased gradually. At no time should the exercise be so strenuous as to inhibit your ability to talk while doing it, i.e., you should not be short of breath either during or after the exercises. One way to monitor precisely the exercise effect on your body is to take your pulse during the exercise. If your heart rate is above 120 beats per minute, you should slow down. (See Glossary for instructions on how to measure your pulse.)

For the pregnant woman on bedrest, options for exercise are somewhat limited, but it may be even more important to exercise in this situation than in a pregnancy without restrictions. With bedrest, if no exercise is performed the muscles become very weak and actual loss of muscle mass can occur (sometimes accounting for weight loss in the pregnant woman despite good nutrition and growth of the fetus). In order to prevent this weakening, and to help the body adjust to the cardiovascular changes in pregnancy, we have designed an exercise program for the pregnant woman on bedrest. For convenience, we have divided the exercises into two groups: for those pregnant women on complete bedrest, and for those on limited activity (e.g., up one hour twice a day). However, before embarking on any of the exercises, please *check with your obstetric practitioner* to be sure the exercises are appropriate for you. (Bring this book with you so that the exercises can be specifically reviewed.)

It is helpful to do the exercise program at a regular time each day (e.g., twenty minutes in the morning and again in the afternoon). Adding music while exercising can help make each session different. Use an exercise log to keep track of your progress in the number of exercises done. If at any time during the exercises you feel uncomfortable, or if you feel an increase in the number of uterine contractions, stop doing the exercises until you check with your practitioner. If you are on medication for premature labor, you need to be especially aware about any shortness of breath or chest pain, and should be sure that your heart rate does not exceed 120 beats per minute at any time. A cassette tape is available (see back of book) to guide you through the exercises at home.

EXERCISES FOR THE PREGNANT WOMAN ON COMPLETE BEDREST

Each part of the body except the abdominal muscles can be gently exercised even if you are on complete bedrest. It is often helpful to begin the daily exercise routine with ten deep inhalations/exhalations held to ten seconds apiece. This breathing exercise strengthens the chest wall muscles. Then begin isometric exercises with each muscle group of the body, except the abdominal muscles. Tighten and loosen each muscle group of the body: face, neck, back, shoulders, arms, hands, thighs, calves, and feet. After the isometric exercises are completed, loosen up each set of joints (e.g., rolling the shoulders in circles). Then follow the next set of exercises designed to strengthen the neck, the arms, the legs, the back, and the pelvis.

Neck and Shoulders

1. Tilt your head to the left as far as possible without strain, keeping shoulders level and relaxed; then to right side. Repeat ten times with each side.

2. Keeping your shoulders level and relaxed, place your left hand on your left cheek, pushing gently with your hand while resisting slightly with your cheek. Turn your head as far to right with this action as possible without strain. Then reverse and use your right hand and your right cheek. Repeat ten times on each side.

3. Raise your left shoulder toward your left ear as far as possible without lifting your head, then relax your shoulder completely and drop. Switch to right side. Repeat two sets of ten with each side.

4. Roll both shoulders up and forward as high and as forward as possible, then reverse. Do six times each way.

Chest and Arms

1. Lift your arms at right angles to your chest at nipple height. Bending your arms, press your palms together firmly. Push together and relax. Do two sets of ten.

2. Extend your arms fully at about shoulder level, using either very light weights or canned goods of the same weight. With your arms still extended, lift your arms slowly over your chest at nipple level, then back down toward the bed slowly. Repeat one to two sets of ten.

3. Still with your arms extended at your sides, using the above weights with your upper arm resting on the bed, bend your arm at the elbow, bringing your hand to the shoulder, working the biceps. Repeat at least two sets of ten.

4. Extending your arms as above, hold weights in your hands, resting the extended arm on the bed. Bend the arm at the wrist, bringing the hand toward the forearm as far as possible, holding the weights in the hand. Do one to two sets of ten, focusing on the forearms.

5. Use a hand grip, available at sporting goods stores, or use a hard rubber ball, tennis ball, or racquetball. Squeeze as tightly as possible, and

you will build up your forearms. Be careful not to unconsciously tighten your abdominal muscles at the same time.

6. Raise each arm and do wrist circles in each direction several times.

Legs and Buttocks

1. Turn on your left side, then roll slightly forward onto your abdomen as far as is comfortable, supporting your weight with the right arm. Lift your right thigh off the bed slightly, focusing on tightening the buttock. Then bend your leg at the knee, with your thigh still off the bed, bringing the heel toward your buttock slowly, then fully extending the leg out. Hold for two seconds extended, then repeat, bringing your heel to your buttock again. Do one set of ten at first, building to two to three sets of ten. Repeat on your right side.

2. Turn on your left side, supporting your body with your right arm, and do leg lifts, lifting your leg straight up from the side with the foot flexed, pointing your toe slightly downward. Do two sets of ten. Repeat on the right side.

3. On your side, lift your leg in the air and do ankle circles. This is good for calf muscles. Repeat on the opposite side.

4. On your back, bend your left knee, bring your thigh to your abdomen, and then extend your left leg. Repeat several times. Repeat with your right leg.

Pelvic and Back Exercises

1. Kegel exercises are designed to strengthen the muscles surrounding the bladder and the vagina, both of which are stretched during the normal course of pregnancy. These exercises are useful both before and after the birth. To do the Kegel exercises, tighten the muscles around the vagina, and hold them tightly for three to five seconds. Release. Repeat between twenty and a hundred times per day. To be sure that you are doing the exercise properly, try to stop the stream of urine when urinating. If you are successful, you are tightening the pelvic floor muscles in the right place.

2. Pelvic tilt exercises are important in keeping the muscles in the lower back strong. You can do these exercises either lying on your back or in knee-chest position facing the floor. Bring the small of your back in

toward your pelvic area as tightly as possible. Hold for ten seconds then thrust it outwards and hold for ten seconds. Repeat. Do this exercise ten to forty times per day.

EXERCISES FOR THE PREGNANT WOMAN WITH LIMITED ACTIVITY

Begin with the exercises above, while you are on the bedrest portion of the day. Then gradually add the following exercises, being sure to check with your obstetrical practitioner, as they involve fifteen to twenty minutes of sitting or standing.

1. In a comfortable sitting position on a small firm pillow, stretch the crown of your head toward the ceiling. Let your head drop back. Allow your mouth to fall open. Now stretch your lower jaw toward the ceiling, and pull your lower lip over the upper one. Relax your jaw, then repeat slowly six to eight times. Return your head to a balanced position with the crown to the ceiling. With your spine thus extended, tuck your chin into the little pocket right above your left shoulder. Interlace your fingers, place them on top of your skull, bring your elbows close together, and allow the weight of your arms to give a steady stretch to the muscles along the back of your neck and down your spine. Hold this position for twenty seconds and concentrate on your breathing. Make it a relaxed flow of air in and out. Repeat with the right shoulder. Then lift your head with the crown extended toward the ceiling again. Turn your head to the right and to the left, with measured breathing. While facing straight ahead, lift up your shoulders toward your ears and drop them. Repeat several times.

2. In a sitting position, with legs out front, extend the crown of the head toward the ceiling. Alternately, gently bend and straighten the right and left knees. When straightening, stretch your heel away and pull your toes toward your body. Press down on each thigh as you repeat this exercise, to provide some resistance and increase the strength of the thigh muscles.

3. While sitting, exhale, and bring the arms together in front of your chest. Inhale, and open them wide. Keep your elbows level with your shoulders. Repeat.

4. In a sitting position, inhale, and open your arms with your elbows bent, then swing your arms open and all the way back. Exhale, and cross them in front of the chest again. Repeat.

5. Stand with your feet parallel and together on a thick book with the heels stretched over the edge. Face the wall and place your hands on a doorknob or against the wall for balance. Come up on your toes. Lower the heels until they go below the edge of the book. Come way up on the toes again, then lower the heels a little farther. Repeat. Exhale, and go up. Inhale and go down.

SUMMARY

After you have completed your exercise program, it is very important to relax. Lie down in the Trendelenburg position (to counteract any possible movement of the fetus downward in the pelvis during the exercising), and do the relaxation breathing suggested in Chapter Eight. After the relaxation exercises are completed, drink a large glass of water or juice.

If you are on limited activity, ask your obstetric practitioner about the possibility of swimming two to three times a week. The water supports the body in a horizontal position, and all of the muscles of the body can be exercised. Swimming is particularly helpful for someone with back problems in pregnancy. Call around to inquire about a pool nearest to you (YWCA, YMCA, community college, or university).

As you approach your thirty-seventh week of pregnancy, think about an exercise program that will help you regain your strength in anticipation of the labor and birth, and the resumption of a very busy schedule once the baby is born. A typical schedule at thirty-seven or thirty-eight weeks might include: swimming every day, twenty-minute walks twice a day, a regular prenatal exercise class twice weekly (a program that includes a postpartum class as well), and a continuation of the exercises that you had been doing the last few months. It is important to work up to this level and to realize that you are still going to need a one- to three-hour rest period each day, even after you are allowed up at thirty-eight weeks without restrictions. The body needs time to recover from the weeks or months of bedrest. You may find that you are particularly weak, even a little dizzy, for the first few days you are up. This will pass in a few days. It is important to honor your body's signals to rest, as weak muscles are easily injured.

After the birth, it is important to continue your exercise program. Many postpartum exercise classes have facilities so that you can bring the baby to class with you (although most pediatricians recommend that the baby not be out and about for approximately a month). It is important to plan on some help at home after the birth, as you will be recovering not only from the labor and delivery, but also from months of bedrest. Back problems are not uncommon in new mothers, and women who experience bedrest for premature labor are especially at risk for this. Not only does the bedrest weaken your back muscles before you resume normal activity at thirty-seven to thirty-eight weeks, but also you suddenly have a lot of additional weight "out front." These changes put special strain on your back muscles. The exercises described here, some help at home, a changing table for the baby at standing height, and a liberal amount of rest (sleep when the baby sleeps), will help prevent postpartum back problems.

BRITTA'S STORY

I was forty-five years old when I became pregnant for the first time. I was in excellent health: mountain climbing, parachuting, jogging. In my pregnancy, I was climbing twenty sets of stairs three to four times a day, and had a sense that no matter what happened during the pregnancy or labor, I was physically ready for it. So to find out that I was in premature labor (precipitated by an automobile accident at thirty-two weeks of pregnancy), was a real shocker. I was hospitalized for twenty-four hours following the initial diagnosis, and was then on bedrest for five weeks.

The worst thing about the bedrest treatment was the inactivity. I went from intense physical activity to zero mobility in a day. In a week the big muscles in my thighs were hurting from the lack of use, which kept me awake at night. My clinicians helped me to devise some safe exercises for bedrest. I would lie on my slantboard doing funny leg raises that didn't use the abdominal muscles. I would do these exercises at all hours until I could sleep. I also had Kevin, my partner, get me some weights for my arms and hands; I actually developed those muscles nicely! As time went on, our daughter's condition seemed more stable, and my physicians suggested swimming. I am basically a drowner, but I swam and loved the exercise in the pool. The change of scene was great! The support of the water for all of my body parts made me feel secure—I didn't feel her pressure on my pelvic floor.

I worried about my work as well. I am an aerospace engineer. I was concerned about the effect my disability leave would have on my career. I was determined not to slip backward in my career after all my hard work. So after my premature labor had stabilized, I was able to go to work (via the back seat of a taxi, as I lay down) for one to two half-days a week. In that manner, I was able to continue to supervise the projects assigned to me, and to be sure that my customers were well taken care of. If I started feeling pelvic pressure once I was at work, especially if accompanied by contractions, I would call it a day and go home early. Once I reached thirty-seven weeks of pregnancy, I was able to return to work half time for three additional weeks, which helped to square away anticipated problems for my eight weeks of maternity leave.

Kevin made me feel as if I never faced the situation alone. We worked as a team: Kevin ran the house and I kept our daughter safe inside my womb. At times it was hard, but Kevin and I were very close. We often had long conversations with our daughter while Kevin put his head on my tummy.

The weekly trips to our doctors had a great effect on our morale. If the cervix was more normal, we felt a positive sense of accomplishment, like we had finished a major successful project. If the exam showed that the cervix was the same or worse, we'd feel down, but usually more determined. Our doctors were always honest with us—but very gentle. That let us trust them, both as to the facts and with our emotions.

Our doctors had set a date when it was "safe for her to come," when she was "big enough." Every indication that she was bigger or longer, every day that passed uneventfully, was a little victory for us. When we reached thirty-eight weeks of pregnancy, it was a celebration—when that day came we knew, all three of us, that "we had done it!"

My labor was very long, a total of four days. At the end of the labor, our baby had some mild fetal distress, and my obstetrician used a vacuum cup on her head to help her through the birth canal. I will always wonder whether if I had been more active during my pregnancy, I would have been able to have a shorter and more manageable labor.

I am so glad that the bedrest is over. I am healthy and ready to resume full exercise. Our daughter Ciren was born at term without needing a Cesarean section, which I had been concerned about, since it represented risks for me. And next week I return to work on a limited basis.

Britta Lindgren, mother of
Ciren (two months).

10

EMBRACING THE CHALLENGE

by Jan Berlin, Ph.D.

> *Our humanity and compassion are born in myriad ways:*
> *at one level through shock, at another through ecstasy*
> *and love.* [1]

When you first became pregnant, you inevitably projected yourself forward in time to imagine what the ensuing months would bring. The
prospect of premature labor was probably not a part of your vision. Even
when individuals have occasion, at the outset of their pregnancy, to be
concerned about a weakened cervix or early labor, they usually think positively and hope that their pregnancy will reach term without incident.

And so the news of preterm labor or weakened cervix comes as a
shock. The prospect of partial or complete bedrest, the chance of hospitalization, the use of medication, the frightening uncertainty, and the dramatic change in the roles you must play during this time all demand one
primary skill: you have to learn to cope! The focus of this book so far has
therefore been about coping—with the medical realities, the time pressures, the stresses, the physiological concerns, and the relationship issues
that inevitably arise during this time.

There is, however, another perspective that must be addressed before
we conclude: the perspective implicit in Dorothy Norman's words. In

---

[1] Norman, Dorothy. *The Hero: Myth/Image/Symbol.* New York: New American
Library, 1969.

essence, we are all heroes in our own life journey. Each of us must face challenges and adversity throughout our lives. And each of us is variously prepared with resources—both internal and external—upon which we can draw to handle these situations as they occur. Such times offer us opportunities to expand our awareness of ourselves and of each other, to deepen our level of humanity and compassion through the suffering and the triumphs that these experiences must bring.

Premature labor is such an experience. The challenge is to allow it to serve as a vehicle for our own growth. Certainly there are times when this road is a difficult one. You have had to substantially alter your life's daily patterns. You have assumed additional financial burdens, you have tolerated weeks or months of medical uncertainty, you have experienced the disruption of nearly every aspect of your life. The process itself can be hard, frustrating, and at times exhausting. And yet this can be an awakening process as well. You don't have to be a victim of premature labor. Instead, the more creative you are in embracing this challenge, the more fully you can derive a feeling of satisfaction from what you and your partner have been able to achieve together. One premature labor partner puts it this way:

> *I would never choose to go through this experience again! But we've come through feeling closer than ever, and now the "increased responsibilities" of caring for our newborn feel like a breeze. Maybe even more importantly, we find that, now that he is here, we don't take our baby so much for granted. And we both know that if we could get through this one, we can probably handle just about anything else as well.*

This emergent sense of confidence and intimacy is typical of many premature labor patients who have chosen to participate actively in the process of sustaining their pregnancies.

Despite the difficulties of this time, you may already be able to recognize ways in which you have creatively embraced the premature labor experience. Perhaps you now have some private jokes or humorous incidents that will remain as enduring memories of this time. There may already be some noticeable shifts in how you have come to feel about yourself, your partner, and your child. Through it all, it becomes increasingly important to remember that all of your efforts, all of your concerns, all of your careful planning and loving diligence have been directed toward your successful participation in one of nature's most miraculous acts of creation: the birth of your child. Recognizing this, we begin the present chapter in the spirit of celebration, saluting all that you both bring to your pregnancy process as co-creators of the child that lives and grows within the womb even as you read these words. We hope that the exercises and techniques presented herein will offer you additional tools for embracing the challenge of premature labor and a weakened cervix in an increasingly creative manner. By using these tools, you too can emerge victorious as the hero of your own life story.

We are all creators in some respects. We all have access to creative potential within ourselves: Creating a meal. Creating a work of art. Creating financial stability. Creating a social event. Creating stillness. Creating a relationship. Creating a child. Silvano Arieti, world-renowned psychiatrist, calls this process the "magic synthesis," for it involves the bringing together of seemingly disparate objects or events toward the creation of something totally new, something that had not been present before. On the pages to follow, we shall focus on this magic synthesis, inviting you to participate actively in exercises and experiences designed to enhance your awareness of your own creative potential during this time of premature labor. Through active sharing, relaxation, and visualization you can learn to further establish a creative alliance within yourself, with your partner, and with your unborn child. In so doing, you can find yourselves developing a growing awareness that this period of your lives, though fraught with difficulties and uncertainties and fears, is filled as well with an opportunity to rally your resources and to experience new levels of creativity together.

CREATING CHALLENGE FROM ADVERSITY

In a recent article, the *Los Angeles Times* reported the story of an ex-policeman who has fulfilled a lifelong dream of becoming an obstetrician. Although he had always wanted to be a physician, this man did not believe he had the intelligence to make it through medical school. Instead, he joined the police force, deciding that this could be another way that he could be of service to humankind. He expected to make police work his lifelong career. It probably would have been, except for the fateful day that he was shot while pursuing a suspect. He survived the injury, but was told he would never be able to resume active duty again. Suddenly his life was in disarray. He had a family to support and many years of professional life before him. The prospect of "early retirement" was unsettling. And then he remembered his dream of becoming a doctor. Despite the fact that his age made him unacceptable to most medical school admissions committees in this country, he persevered. He gained admission at the University of the Philippines. And he excelled. He now is completing his medical residency, and he plans to practice obstetrics and gynecology when he is finished.

Unwilling to be a victim of his life circumstances, this man took the bull by the horns and turned a dream into a reality. This is the essence of creating challenge from adversity. What is important is not only the course of action that you decide to take, but also the attitude with which you view the adverse condition itself. The more you can maintain a positive but realistic attitude, and the more you can identify the self-affirming opportunities inherent in any life experience, the better prepared you will be to embrace the challenge itself. The next two exercises will help you to achieve these goals.

Developing Positive Self-Talk

Self-talk is a term from cognitive psychology referring to the words and phrases we say to ourselves. Positive self-talk usually takes the form of congratulatory statements (e.g., "I did a really good job on that project") or optimistic phrases (e.g., "I know everything will be all right"). Negative self-talk includes self-deprecatory comments ("I never do anything right"), guilt-inducing phrases ("I ought to be ashamed of myself for making my partner work so hard"), pessimistic predictions ("My cervix will probably efface even more by next week"), or just plain giving up.

Psychological research has shown that negative self-talk can erode self-confidence, increase stress, cause us to feel depressed, and block access to our natural coping resources. Positive self-talk, on the other hand, can bolster our confidence, elevate our mood, provide a healthy frame of mind from which to plan a course of action, and enable us to face challenges more effectively. Nevertheless, we all fall into negative self-talk patterns from time to time. The purpose of this exercise is to learn to identify our negative self-talk and replace it with positive phrases.

To begin, we have listed several statements that are typically made by couples in premature labor. For the first three, we show you how a negative self-statement can be transformed into a positive one. The remaining negative statements are for you to transform yourselves. You and your partner might want to work on the list separately and then compare notes. In this way, you will find that there are many ways to transform a negative statement into a positive one. As long as your transformed sentence is realistic, positive, and affirms your ability to handle the situation before you, it qualifies as positive self-talk.

Negative Self-Statement	*Positive Self-Statement*
"This bedrest is never going to end."	"I'm in my thirtieth week now, so I just have seven weeks to go. It's a long time and sometimes very frustrating, but there is an end in sight and I know I'm going to make it."
"I'll never be able to pay all these bills."	"I've got a lot more bills to pay than I expected. But I know that I can sit down and figure out a financial strategy to be sure we will make out okay."
"There's nothing I can do now—it's all up to the doctors."	"There *are* ways that I can be an active participant in this premature labor process."

Now you try a few:

Negative Self-Statement	*Positive Self-Statement*
"I'm a mess—I don't even know what's happening in my own household!"	
"My poor partner—I'm not doing nearly enough to keep things happy."	
"If I were a better partner, this wouldn't be happening."	

Negative Self-Statement	*Positive Self-Statement*
"All this medication is probably do-ing terrible things to our child—what kind of parent am I!"	
"My partner probably hates me for having to go through this."	
"Nobody's called today—they're probably all sick of me."	

Now that you have had a chance to practice on the above phrases, be mindful of your own self-talk throughout the day. If you're the woman on bedrest, you might want to jot down any negative self-statements and then transform them into positive phrases, just as you did above. Partners can do this as a mental exercise, perhaps while driving in the car or during meal preparation times. By sharing some of these phrases with each other, you can begin to reinforce those thoughts that shed a positive light on your handling of this experience.

As with any other difficult period, premature labor does not have to erode the intimacy between you and your partner. In fact, it may provide fertile ground for stating your acceptance of and confidence in yourself and in your partner. The above exercise achieves this by addressing what you say to yourself. The next exercise, to be done with your partner, deals with what you say to one another.

Recognizing Your Co-Creations

In all likelihood, your first act of co-creation together was the formation of your bond of love, a bond whose manifestation you now celebrate in the form of this pregnancy. So take a moment, and think back to your rela-tionship's beginnings. Discuss together where you first met and what ini-tially attracted you to one another. Think about the course of your early months together. Inevitably, there were wonderful moments and difficult moments, easy times and challenging times, special memories that forged the character of who you are together. On separate pieces of paper, note some of those moments, some of those challenges. Now share what you have written. Are there similarities in your lists? Differences? Spend some time thinking about the challenges. How did you deal with them at that time? On what resources did you draw? In retrospect, what opportunities did these challenges provide you that you otherwise might have missed?

Coming through these challenges usually strengthens a relationship and deepens the connection between you.

Now focus your attention on this pregnancy. Be open to the viewpoint that this is yet another challenge that you face together, a challenge to draw upon all of your inner resources and to focus those resources in a concerted way. In so doing, you deepen your own bond as well as the new bond you are creating with your unborn child. Take some time to review together how, individually and as a couple, you have faced this present challenge. What resources are you using? How are you getting the support you need from within yourself and from each other? Placing yourself in your partner's role, imagine what it must be like in the other position. Notice how different your partner's challenges are from your own. And finally, voice your appreciation for (a) how your partner has been coping with the challenges of the premature labor experience; and (b) what you can recognize as your partner's support of your role during this time.

This exercise may generate some feelings between you as you explore these issues. If the feelings are positive, be sure to share them . . . that's part of the payoff for revealing yourselves to each other! If the feelings are negative or conflicted, this may be an opportunity to do some constructive problem solving for both of you. While lack of communication can keep the premature labor experience stuck at the level of adversity, sorting out your differences in a loving manner can spark a renewed sense of intimacy between you.

TAPPING INNER RESOURCES THROUGH VISUALIZATION

During the Hermetic period in ancient Egypt, it was believed that the images held in one's thoughts created a powerful influence both on the material world and on one's attitudes and behaviors. This belief prompted that ancient civilization to incorporate visualization techniques designed to have a positive impact on one's life. For example, a soldier besieged with fear would be told to close his eyes and imagine himself to be a great warrior engaged safely and victoriously in battle, thereby transforming his fear into courage. Farmers ritualistically pictured abundant crops, and healers invoked images of their patients free of illness and disease.

During the past twenty years, a resurgence of interest in the use of imagery techniques has swept this country. Athletes now use imagery, and report noticeable improvements in their performance as a result of incorporating this technique. Schools that implement visualization exercises to stimulate creative thinking report that students are more enthusiastically involved and that writing skills have markedly improved. Corporations have introduced these techniques as part of management training, and a host of workshops and materials offered across the country attest to the growing popularity of this concept among the public at large.

In a clinical setting, psychologists and physicians have also begun using imagery techniques for a variety of problems. Not unlike the imagery used in the ancient Egyptian civilization, these techniques rely upon the visualizer's ability to become absorbed in an inner life experience, sometimes called a waking dream, to effect certain desired changes in psychological and physical states. Depending upon the nature of the image, these visualizations can enhance performance, shed light on psychosomatic concerns, or simply provide the visualizer with respite from the exigencies of the everyday world.

Sometimes the changes that result from imagery are quite rapid, stimulated by a sudden impact from a single image. An actor who had been using imagery to aid in memorizing a long part suddenly saw the image of a juggler twirling a plate on the end of a long pole. As he watched with fascination, he realized that what enabled the juggler to perform this feat was his capacity to maintain a unitary focus for long periods of time. With delight, the actor reported that this had clearly been his problem with memorizing the script . . . he had simply been concentrating on too many different things at once to make the lines his own. This sudden awareness enabled him to redirect his efforts. Within a matter of days, he had mastered the part.

At other times, changes produced by imagery take longer to manifest and seem to be the product of an ongoing process in which unconscious mechanisms are activated and channeled on the patient's behalf. A case example illustrates this:

A woman in her early thirties who had been suffering with an extreme case of eczema (a skin reaction similar to an allergy) since age fourteen was referred for treatment by her dermatologist. She had been only minimally responsive to traditional medical interventions, and viewed the imagery work as a last resort.

In the early phases of treatment, the patient would imagine herself on a special, private beach. She would lie on the sand and picture a radiant sun spreading warmth throughout her body and healing the eczematic sores. She would then see herself enter the ocean and watch as the gentle waves washed away any evidence of eczema, leaving her skin fresh and clear.

While the imagery was vivid and relaxing, it caused no change in the patient's skin condition. One day, rather than going to the beach, the patient found herself at the top of a ski slope with a very close friend. Together they skied down the mountain, marveling at the beauty of the freshly fallen snow. On the way back, the patient saw a lone figure making its way toward them. She paused with her friend and waited as an old man with white hair and a rumpled shirt approached. When he reached the two women, he began to talk to them about a friend of theirs who had died the year before [this event had actually happened in the patient's life]. Upon mention of the deceased friend, the woman who had accompanied the patient down the ski slope began to weep, but the patient herself remained stoic. With compassion in his voice, the old man said to the patient, "My dear, as long as you refuse to allow the tears to fall from your eyes, they will continue to come out of your skin." This profound insight, not atypical in imagery experiences of this kind, made quite an impression on the patient. Yet still there was no change in her skin condition.

In a subsequent session approximately six weeks later, the patient returned from the healing beach only to report the presence of an intense headache that she had not had prior to the imagery experience. She decided to go back into the image to see if she could understand what might have caused the headache. When the patient returned to the beach, she noticed a stereo amplifier with the volume set at ten. She immediately understood this as representing the intensity of her headache. Walking further, she came upon a barn. Inside were several horses in stalls. One particular horse captured her interest. Named Bonnet, this horse was chained within its stall. The patient, upset by the chains, went to find the stable master to get permission to release the horse. When she found him, he turned out to be the *same old man* whom she had encountered on the ski slopes weeks before. He told her that she certainly could release Bonnet from her chains.

Pleased, the patient returned to the barn, unlatched the locks, and let Bonnet go free. She watched as Bonnet ran out of the barn and disappeared over the horizon. On the way back, the patient passed the stereo amplifier and noted that the volume was now set at zero. When she returned to the waking state, her headache was gone. And as of the next week, her eczematic symptoms began to disappear.

This case example illustrates several important features of the imagery process. First, there are times when we receive in imagery information that is previously unknown to us and that can be potentially catalytic for our own growth. This information sometimes is delivered by other characters in the image, such as the old man in the above example. These "guides," as they are often called, can be rich sources of support and insight, and usually can be contacted in subsequent imagery experiences. Second, the imagery often unfolds like a children's story, drawing upon symbols and appealing to the child within each of us. It is, for some people, a process much like a dream. However, in contrast to the dream state in which we are basically passive observers, imagery permits far more interaction with the conscious self. Thus we experience elements of choice, direction, and interaction in the image that are qualitatively different from the dream state.

Each person visualizes differently. Some people see pictures in their mind's eye that are every bit as vivid and colorful as the images projected on a television screen. Others visualize in a disjointed fashion, seeing a series of disconnected pictures that they then tie together to provide some thematic understanding of the message contained within the image. Still others report that their images are vague and diffuse, and it is more the thought of the image than the image itself that guides them through the visualization experience. To discover your own distinctive way of visualizing, close your eyes and think about an orange. See if you can picture it in your mind's eye. Now imagine that you are holding it in your hand. Can you feel the roughness of the skin? Peel the orange. As the juices squirt, you may be able to smell and taste the fruit itself. Now open your eyes.

This experience was designed to test your multi-sensory capacity for imagery. How many senses were you able to involve? Were some senses easier than others? While most people find that visualizing an image is easier than evoking other senses such as taste or smell, others who report no capacity to produce visual images are able to have full access to images through other sensory modalities.

Generally, your capacity to use imagery will improve with practice. We encourage you to do so, not only with the following exercises but with your own self-initiated experiences as well (sometimes it's fun just to close your eyes and see what images spontaneously come to mind!).

The exercises that we have included here have been developed specifically for the preterm labor patient and her partner. Most of these exercises are done in a relaxed position, with eyes closed, so that your imagination may wander freely with the images suggested. To facilitate your fullest participation you may want to do one of two things:

1. Dictate the text of the imagery into a tape recorder and then use your own taped voice as a guide for the experience itself;

2. Take turns with your partner, acting as guides for each other.

In either case, be sure to speak slowly and *allow plenty of time* to explore the images fully. Silences pass much more quickly when you are doing imagery than when you are in a waking state, and you may find that you need to adjust your pauses accordingly to allow sufficient time to experience all the images that come to mind.

Before starting a visualization exercise, position yourself in a comfortable place (usually a bed, couch, or comfortable armchair are ideal) where you can be uninterrupted for fifteen to twenty minutes. If you are a premature labor partner, you might want to check first with your partner on bedrest so that you can respond to any of her needs before you get started. It is helpful to unplug the phone as well, so you won't be startled by a sudden ring.

When you are ready to begin, uncross your arms and legs, take a deep breath, and close your eyes. Using either the tape or your partner's voice as a guide, you can begin to picture the suggested scenes in your mind's eye. From time to time, you may encounter people or animals or other mythological figures in your imagery. If this occurs, feel free to interact with them in the image. You may find that these various characters can function as guides for you, much like the white-haired old man in the example cited earlier. You can feel free to ask these guide figures whatever questions you'd like, including questions of clarification about the visualization experience itself (use the same kind of "internal voice" that you use when talking to yourself). You may find that these guides can soon become allies in this internal environment, shedding light on your current situation, offering support, and generally being available to you whenever you enter this imaginary realm.

When you are ready to return to a full waking state, you can simply suggest to yourself that the image you have been seeing will gradually begin to fade away. As it does so, simply return your awareness to your room, to the feeling of your body on the bed or couch or chair, and to the sounds of your external environment. Very gradually, count backwards silently to yourself from ten to one. By the time you reach the number one, your eyes will come open and you will be fully awake and alert.

The Meadow

Make yourself comfortable, take a deep breath, and close your eyes. See yourself in a meadow. It may be a meadow that you've visited before, or perhaps a totally new place. Either way, take some time to get to know this meadow. (Pause.) Notice any sounds in the meadow, such as the chirping of birds or the sound of a breeze rustling the leaves of a tree. Be aware of where you are, and how you're feeling, and what kind of day it is. [If you are the partner conducting this image, give the imager a chance to respond verbally to these perceptions. You may want to offer assurances that speech will come very easily without in any way interrupting their internal focus.] In time, you will come upon a shovel. Allow the shovel to guide you to some place in the meadow where you can begin to dig. You will find that under the surface of the meadow are all kinds of objects for your discovery. See what you dig up today. (Long pause. Let the imager describe what appears). If you have discovered more than one object, choose one that particularly captures your interest. (Pause.) Now allow this object to carry you up and out of the meadow, to a totally new place where you can gain additional insights about the meaning of the object you have found and its potential contribution to your own growth at this time. (Long pause.)

Take as long as you'd like in this new place. When you have finished, let the object carry you back to the meadow. (Pause.) Take some time to be in this meadow once more, feeling its tranquility and knowing that you can return there as often as you'd like. When you are ready, gradually bring yourself all the way back to a full waking state, feeling relaxed and refreshed and remembering as much or as little of this experience as you would like.

The Healing Stream

Take three breaths, breathing in a gentle blue light and breathing out any tension or negativity that might block your full and deep relaxation.

See yourself walking along a path in the woods. As you make your way, you begin to hear the sounds of a babbling brook or stream. Follow the sounds until you reach the stream. (Pause.) On the bank of the stream, you find a cup. Dipping the cup into the stream, fill it with water and bring it to your lips. Gently taste the water, feeling its invigorating and refreshing effects as it enters your system. (Pause.) Know that the waters of this stream are healing waters, providing your body with whatever it needs to feel healthy and to function in an optimal way.

For pregnant women: Allow the gentleness of these healing waters to soothe your abdominal area, spreading throughout your body a peaceful feeling of restfulness and quiet. Know that your child is experiencing this peacefulness, as are you. Together, feel the reverie of this spot along the bank of the stream. Remain here for as long as you'd like, lulled by the sound of these soothing waters and comforted by the gentleness of this place.

For partners: Feel these healing waters enliven you and replenish all of your bodily resources. Feel an increase of energy as you allow the water to pass through your system, providing much needed rest and rejuvenation to all of the cells of your body. Draw another long, cool drink, and sense your readiness to resume your daily activities, feeling bright and alert and clear. Know that you can return to this stream whenever you'd like, to provide yourself with a much-deserved rest and to fuel your resources with the invigoration of this stream.

Creating Stillness

This exercise offers the pregnant woman a different method by which to quiet the body. It may be particularly useful at those times when your mind is racing, or when you feel antsy from inactivity, or when you have an overwhelming drive to resume your normal activity level even though you know that you can't. For partners of premature labor patients, this exercise may provide you with a means by which to take a break from the whirlwind pace and endless stream of activity that has become so much a part of your life.

To begin, settle into a comfortable posture and close your eyes. Take three deep breaths, feeling all the tension in your body flowing out with each exhalation. As you breathe out the third time, begin to focus more and more deeply on your own inner darkness. Picture yourself gradually floating deeper and deeper, like a feather in a canyon, drifting deeper and deeper within yourself. (Pause.) Now become the feather. Feel yourself, without effort, gently making your way downward to the floor of the canyon. (Pause.) Breathe out, and gently touch down. See yourself in a vast natural cathedral, ringed with mountains. The day is clear; the air is still. Notice the feeling of profound quiet all around you. (Long pause.) Breathe out, and know in this place of stillness a deep inner peacefulness. A freedom from anxiety and concerns. A feeling of being far, far away, alone with yourself and [for expectant mothers] with the child who grows within you. Notice the quiet, rhythmic pattern of your breathing and the complete relaxation of the body as you rest peacefully here on the canyon floor. From this deep inner place, you can reflect upon the following words of wisdom from an ancient Chinese text:

> *Empty yourself of everything.*
> *Let the mind rest at peace.*
> *The ten thousand things rise and fall*
> *   while the Self watches their return.*
> *They grow and flourish and then return*
> *   to the source.*
> *Returning to the source is stillness,*
> *   which is the way of nature.* [2]
>
> Lao-tzu
> from **Tao Te Ching**

Take as long as you want to be with this "way of nature." You may find yourself visually continuing to see the image of the canyon. Or alternatively, you may find that that image fades away and you settle into a deep, amorphous, and sometimes vast experience of a void where thoughts and images come and go. Here the overriding sense is one of formlessness and timelessness and deep inner quiet. Either way, you can remain in this state for as long as you want. When you feel finished, breathe out once more and make your return very gradually all the way back to an awareness of the everyday world and your everyday life experience. Bring with you all of this inner quiet and peacefulness as you continue to meet the challenge of stillness and rest [for the expectant mother] or of centeredness and enhanced capacity for activity [for the partner].

Finding a Special Place

Couples in premature labor have found that it can be very helpful to have a special place in imagery where they can go together or separately to be with themselves and with the process of holding on. This visualization experience is designed to facilitate the creation of that special place. As such, it might be particularly appropriate for partners to guide one another through this exercise, using the text to follow.

---

[2] Lao-tzu. *Tao Te Ching*. Translated by Jane English and Gia-Fu Feng. New York: Vintage Books, 1972.

When the expectant mother is visualizing, it will be important to help her select a special place that encourages, both symbolically and physiologically, a still uterus. Avoid such places as a pounding ocean surf or a rushing river. Images of water such as this may evoke a response from the "internal waters" of the body. One woman, for example, discovered that when she went to the ocean's edge, the feeling of the tide and the undertow pulling into the sea began to promote contractions rather than quiet them. While not everybody is as physiologically responsive to imagery as she was, it is best to pick images that will facilitate your ultimate goal. You may want to select wide, grassy meadows or a deep forest or an interior environment such as a wonderful cottage or a place by a fire in a rustic cabin. Feel free to let your imagination guide you within the guidelines established herein.

Take a moment to relax and get comfortable. As you breathe out three times, give yourself quiet inner permission to use the next period of time to create your own special place, a unique environment ideally suited for your own rest and replenishment.

With your eyes closed, see yourself walking along the outskirts of a forest. As you make your way into the forest, become more and more aware of the sights and sounds and sensations that surround you. As you see yourself in this environment, describe for your partner where you are and how you are feeling. (Long pause.) As you go farther, you come upon a resting place. It could be inside a cottage or cabin, or it may be somewhere outside where you can be comfortable and serene, such as a clearing in the forest, a patch of green grass, or perhaps a nearby cave. Select an insulated, gentle space where you can feel comfort and support. As you find this place, describe it for your partner [if you are being guided] and let yourself get to know it well. (Pause.) This place is your own special setting. You can visit it for relaxation or replenishment, or to be in contact with your child, or simply as a sanctuary from the multitude of tasks that await you in your day-to-day life. Take as long as you like in this place, feeling the replenishment and relaxation and the capacity to provide yourself with all that you need to master the challenges before you. You may want to review in your mind the progress that you've made already, the resources upon which you've drawn, the sense of confidence and certainty that you can and will hold on until that thirty-seventh week, after which your baby, fully grown and healthy, can be born.

You can return to this special place whenever you like, with or without the presence of your partner, simply by closing your eyes, taking a deep breath and picturing once more in your mind's eye this inner setting, and feeling, with as many of the senses as you can call upon, the experience to be had here.

Contacting the Inner Physician

Albert Schweitzer was once asked to explain how tribal shamans were able to effect such remarkable cures without the aid of sophisticated medical knowledge and technology. He replied that these tribal doctors "awakened the inner physician of the patient," thereby promoting the healing from within the patients themselves. Building on this concept, we now invite you to meet your own inner physician, a special type of guide to be encountered in imagery and to be used particularly to facilitate your own involvement with your body's state of wellness.

To begin this image, breathe out three times and see yourself in your own special place. Take some time to relax and center yourself in this place. (Pause.) When you feel ready, close your eyes within the image. Focus only on the breath as it flows through the nostrils. Be mindful of the rise and fall of the chest or abdomen as you breathe. (Pause.) In time, you will feel a gentle nudge or tap on the shoulder. Knowing that your inner physician has arrived, open your eyes. Make contact with your physician with your eyes, and feel the deep and profound connection that you can establish together. (Long pause.) If you would like, feel free to ask your inner physician any questions, including questions about maintaining your body's health and sustaining your pregnancy. Be open to your physician's responses. (Long pause.) Does the inner physician have anything else to share with you at this time? (Pause.) Remain together for as long as you want, continuing to talk or simply sharing silence together. When your visit is complete, make your goodbyes for now, knowing that you can summon your inner physician to this special place whenever you choose.

HOLDING YOUR BABY

As time progresses in your pregnancy and you begin to feel more confident about its outcome, you will probably find that your images of the baby and of yourselves as parents reemerge. We encourage you to enjoy these growing feelings of attachment as a means both of preparing to have a child and of creating closeness with your baby now. Such closeness will help you to feel like a family already working toward a common goal. You may have more quiet time together than does a mobile pregnant couple. This time provides an opportunity for you to tune into your baby and to share this precious time as a family.

The following techniques have been successfully used by other couples to "hold" their baby in utero. Some of these methods you may already have discovered yourself, while others may be new to you.

1. Each place a hand on the woman's abdomen. Feel the baby's movement. Sense whether you can do a dance with the baby, attracting your child to your warmth. Try to feel a foot, knee, or elbow as it protrudes through the uterus. Play with your baby.

2. Hold one another belly to belly and feel the baby's movement. Imagine that you are hugging your child between you so closely that the three of you have merged.

3. Lie quietly again each with one hand on the woman's abdomen and the other hand in your partner's hand. Close your eyes. Breathe deeply three times, relaxing your body with each exhalation. Allow your mind to go blank, emptying it of thoughts from your day. Feel the warmth of your hand in your partner's hand. Imagine the warmth of your other hand radiating through the uterus to the baby. Feel your connection to your child. Feel the circle of warmth created by your partner, yourself, and your baby. Imagine the warmth as a white light bathing the baby and bringing calm to the womb. Tune in to your baby as a person. What impressions do you get about your baby? Appreciate the unique qualities. Appreciate the miracle of growth. Feel your warmth lending strength and shelter to your baby. Experience the warmth between yourself and your partner as white light lending strength to your union. Let the white light surround all of you, and bask in it. When you are ready, return to the room and open your eyes.

Variation: As images or impressions of the baby come to mind, share them with one another to create a shared image.

Embracing your child is a fitting way to conclude this chapter on embracing the challenge of premature labor or weakened cervix. These last exercises may serve as a joyous reminder that a living being—the child of your creation—will soon be your reward for all the effort you are each expending at the present time. Through the use of positive self-talk, visualization, and direct and playful contact with the child within your womb, you may find that you can triumph over the initial shock of your diagnosis.

As the days pass and the moment of birth approaches, your excited anticipation can awaken that other vehicle through which Dorothy Norman tells us that humanity and compassion are born . . . the dimensions of ecstasy and love.

CONCLUSION

by Peggy Henning Berlin, Ph.D.

If you have not done so thus far, we urge you now to take a moment to consider what it is that you are, in truth, doing during these weeks of "holding on." Take some time to imagine that you are able to hover somewhere above a typical daily scene, watching yourself and your partner, your family and friends, while you are lying in bed or carrying out various tasks. Take some time to notice what is occurring from a different perspective, outside of time and space. You can see the relationship between people's various roles, though distant from one another. You can see the relationship between yesterday and today. You may even sense continuity with the future. From such a perspective, the question of what you are "doing"—of what this is all about—has a number of answers on a number of different levels.

The familiar question, "What are you doing with yourself?" prompts one kind of response: "I am reading, watching television, catching up on paperwork." Indeed, the level of daily busy-ness is an integral one. It not only gets things done, it keeps you feeling involved with life, and sane. Perhaps you are accomplishing your daily activities differently now—with more or less efficiency, with a deeper appreciation of those around you. During this period of your life, perhaps more than at any other, you will probably pay attention to what you "do" with time. Because of this, and because of the need to change the way you usually spend time, you have the opportunity to look at yourself, to reflect, and, if you choose, to modify.

On another level, what you are "doing" during these weeks is, of course, protecting your baby. Babies born prematurely simply have less ability to bounce back from early complications or initially weak vital signs. One patient being treated for a weakened cervix relayed to us a story typical of those we hear all too frequently. A friend had just given birth to her second premature baby, this one suffering from severe eye damage resulting from the necessary oxygen treatments. Though her first child had been born prematurely, the friend had not been deemed by her practitioner as being at high risk, nor had her cervix been monitored for change. She then went on to deliver her second premature baby. The patient who related the story was grateful for having had her own weakened cervix diagnosed and treated early, although at times she had wondered whether the treatment was "overreacting." However, in hearing about her friend's baby, and now having her own healthy full-term infant at home, she realized what a small price a few months of bedrest was.

Fortunately this type of story is becoming the exception and not the rule, as the result of medical and public education. With aggressive medical attention, parents have increased opportunities to avert premature birth. Every week that passes with your baby in the womb gives your baby a better chance for health. We hope that while you are endeavoring to do as little as possible (if you're a woman on bedrest) or as much as possible (if you're her partner), this view of what you're *really* doing will help you to keep perspective about the relative importance of other things. Together you are giving your baby the best birthday present possible—time and health.

Finally, there is another level to what you are "doing." From a perspective beyond our daily vision, the present circumstance serves, ironically, as an opportunity for yourselves, for your family, for your child. For each of you there may be opportunities to learn something different, something personally relevant and expanding. It is each person's challenge to recognize, interpret, and accept or reject the experience presented. Some personal anecdotes come to mind.

When I was hospitalized with premature labor at twenty-four weeks in my pregnancy, Jan and I were gently challenged by Patty to consider to what lengths we would wish to go to preserve life should our baby be born. Amid tears and great fear, the image of a prematurely born baby I had once assessed in my psychological practice came to mind. When I had seen her, this baby was eighteen months old with severely debilitating cerebral palsy. She had no use of her limbs or trunk save for her left arm. She did not yet comprehend or use language, but had a sense of herself in the world and in relation to other people that was inspiring. When I greeted her, her entire face lit up with a smile. When placed on her tummy on the floor with a toy in front of her, she used her one good arm to drag her torso the few feet required to get it. This child's spirit and will, her joy in her own accomplishment no matter how small, made me want to lend her anything I could to enable her to do whatever she could. In the moment of my questioning about my own child, the meaning of my encounter with that baby became clearer. It was as though my memory of her spoke for my unborn child, asking me to do all I could for him. What medical decisions we might have made had we been faced with a severely compromised newborn are separate questions I can't answer, having not had to do so. Encountering this baby's memory at that particular moment, however, gave me optimism and purpose.

Other encounters occurred as well. My own mother had lost twins born prematurely when I was a child. The threat of history repeating itself challenged our family to change our usual style of denial where fear is concerned. Whereas earlier I might have understood my mother's withdrawal and allowed it in order to "protect" her from her feelings, this time was different. I needed and wanted my mother's support. The challenge to her was to reencounter her pain in order to acknowledge my need. The challenge to me was first, to believe in my own mother's capacity both to face her own feelings and to support me, and second, to allow myself to depend on others—for me an altogether difficult task.

All life events offer us opportunities, but some of them, such as a complicated pregnancy, really get our attention so that we're compelled to ask, "Now what's this all about?" Chances are it's "about" a lot of things. Only *you* can hear the messages in it for you. It is our sincere hope that this time of "holding on" will be more than *just* "holding on"—more than merely clinging to the status quo while biding time. Rather, we hope it will be a time of embracing: embracing your circumstances, your family and friends, each other, your child, and most of all, embracing the larger-than-life aspects of yourself and your own life's journey.

APPENDIX A

GLOSSARY
OF MEDICAL TERMS

Amniocentesis: the withdrawal of amniotic fluid from around the fetus via a needle inserted through the abdominal wall of the pregnant woman. The fluid is then sent for various tests, such as genetic studies or evaluation of lung maturity. (See Appendix B.)

Amniotic fluid: the fluid surrounding the fetus.

Amniotic sac: the membranes that enclose the fetus in the amniotic fluid. When the amniotic sac breaks, the membranes are considered ruptured (the fluid leaks out through the vagina).

Anemia: a lower-than-normal level of red blood cells in the body. In the adult female, a hemoglobin of 9.0 grams or less signifies a severe anemia. Usually anemia in pregnancy is caused by iron deficiency, which can be corrected by iron supplementation.

Anesthesia: the administration of medication or gases for the relief of pain, in particular during surgery or labor. (See Appendix B.)

Anesthesiologist: a physician who has had special training in the administration of anesthesia.

Apnea: an interruption in the normal breathing pattern, with decreased frequency of respirations.

Betamethasone: a steroid medication occasionally administered to mothers in premature labor in order to accelerate the lung maturity of the fetus.

Bilirubin: a breakdown product of red blood cells that, in excess, can cause jaundice.

BPD: biparietal diameter; a measurement of the fetal head obtained during an ultrasound examination.

Bradley: a type of childbirth education whose formal name is "Husband Coached Childbirth."

Braxton-Hicks contractions: uterine tightenings commonly felt during the course of pregnancy that do not cause cervical change.

Bronchopulmonary dysplasia: a chronic lung disease often associated with prolonged use of the respirator by an infant.

Cerclage: a suture placed in the cervix for the treatment of an incompetent or weakened cervix.

Cervical conization: a surgical procedure in which a portion of the cervix is removed, usually to remove abnormal cells that were found on a Pap smear.

Cervix: the lower part of the uterus that protrudes into the vagina, bounded by the internal os above and the external os below.

Cesarean section: the delivery of a newborn through an incision in the mother's abdomen. A Cesarean section is major surgery and possible risks include bleeding, infection, and injury to the bladder. Having one Cesarean section does not necessarily mean that a woman needs to have them in the future; this depends upon the type of incision in the uterus at the time of the previous Cesarean sections.

Childbirth education classes: classes that prepare the pregnant woman and her partner for the labor and delivery process.

Chorioamnionitis: an infection involving the uterus, the amniotic fluid, and usually the fetus.

Colostrum: the substance expressed from the breasts during the first three days postpartum. Colostrum is composed of rich proteins and is produced specifically for the nourishment of the newborn. The breast milk usually "comes in" on the third day postpartum.

CPR: cardiopulmonary resuscitation, a technique used for revival of an infant or person who has either stopped breathing or whose heart has stopped beating. Often CPR classes are offered at the local American Red Cross or at the YMCA/YWCA.

D&C: dilation and curettage, a minor surgical procedure used to scrape the lining of the uterus, e.g., for an abortion, or for treatment of irregular or prolonged menstrual bleeding.

Demerol: a short-acting narcotic often used to relieve pain during labor.

DES: Diethylstilbesterol, a compound (steroid in nature) given to women in the 1950s and 1960s to prevent miscarriage. This compound is now known to affect the children who were being carried at the time this drug was administered to their mothers. There is a very rare incidence of vaginal cancer in DES daughters; however, a large proportion of these DES daughters have infertility problems and problems related to premature labor or weakened cervix. DES sons may have urological problems that involve various parts of the male reproductive tract.

Dexamethasone: a steroid used to increase fetal lung maturity.

Down's syndrome: a form of moderate retardation that can be detected by amniocentesis, as there is an extra chromosome in the genetic "makeup" of the fetus.

Effacement: thinning out of the uterine cervix.

Epidural: a type of regional anesthesia in which the lower part of the body is numbed by the injection of medication through a needle in the back into the epidural canal. (See Appendix B.)

Episiotomy: a vaginal incision that is used to facilitate the delivery of the baby.

Exchange transfusion: a blood transfusion that is given to a baby who has an extremely high bilirubin level after a small portion of the baby's blood has been withdrawn. The effect of the exchange transfusion is to decrease the total level of bilirubin.

Fern test: a test used to detect rupture of the membranes. A drop of vaginal secretions is placed on a slide, which is evaluated under a microscope. If there is a fern pattern on the slide, amniotic fluid is probably present.

Fetal distress: a situation in which the fetus is not tolerating the labor or the pregnancy well. Fetal distress is usually interpreted by a fetal heart rate tracing (decelerations, flatness of baseline), or a fetal scalp sample that shows low oxygen or an acidotic pH of the fetus.

Fetal scalp sample: a sample of fetal blood to determine the acid-base balance of the baby during labor. The sample is obtained by placing a speculum in the vagina, then making a small "finger-stick" into the scalp and withdrawing a minute portion of the fetal blood. This blood is sent directly to the lab, where it is analyzed in order to see if any fetal distress is present.

Fibroid: a muscle overgrowth in the wall of the uterus, very commonly found in women in their thirties and forties. Women with known fibroids in their uterus have an increased risk of premature labor, intrauterine growth retardation, and placental abruption.

Forceps: spoon-like instruments that can be used to help deliver a baby vaginally, e.g., when (1) the mother is too exhausted to push during the last part of labor, or (2) an immediate delivery is necessary and there is not time to allow the baby to be pushed out by the mother.

Gastric aspirate: a specimen of stomach fluid obtained from the newborn by passing a small feeding tube through the nostril into the stomach cavity. This fluid may be examined for any evidence of inflammation or bacteria, and might be indicative of whether or not the newborn baby has a serious infection.

General anesthesia: anesthesia in which the patient is "put to sleep" by a combination of medications given through an IV and gases administered either by mask or through a tube that is placed in the airway. (S ₃ Appendix B.)

Gestational age: the age in weeks of a fetus, calculated from the first day of the last menstrual period.

Gestational diabetes: the development of diabetes mellitus (hyperglycemia or increased blood sugar) during the course of the pregnancy. This condition occurs in 5 percent of all pregnant women, and usually disappears postpartum. No insulin is required except in rare instances.

Hydrocephalus: increased fluid buildup within the brain due to faulty drainage channels, e.g., as a result of an intracranial hemorrhage blocking the natural flow of the fluid surrounding the brain. A shunt can often be placed in the brain to alleviate this abnormal pressure.

Hypertension: elevation of blood pressure above a normal range.

Hypocalcemia: low calcium level in the blood.

Hypoglycemia: low blood sugar.

Hypothermia: an abnormally low body temperature.

Incompetent cervix: a cervix that is effacing and dilating in the absence of uterine contractions before thirty-seven weeks of gestation.

Intracranial hemorrhage: a hemorrhage into the soft tissues of the brain, which can either resolve spontaneously or, if extensive, can cause brain damage.

Intravenous fluid: salt solutions that are infused through a small catheter in a vein in order to provide hydration. (See Appendix B.)

IUGR: intrauterine growth retardation, a condition in which the fetus does not grow as well as expected. This condition can occur at any time during pregnancy, but is more common in the last three months of pregnancy. Causes of IUGR can be hypertension, placental dysfunction, etc.

Jaundice: "yellow" color of the skin, caused by excess bilirubin products. Jaundice is a very common problem in newborns and is usually easily treated.

Lamaze: a type of prepared childbirth class.

Magnesium sulfate: an intravenous medication that is used to treat premature labor or hypertension present in labor.

Meningitis: an infection in the spinal fluid that is very serious, with possible long-term consequences (e.g., hearing loss).

Metabolic imbalance: an imbalance in the body between acid or base products. This condition can be treated medically.

Monitoring: a recorded observation of both uterine contractions and fetal heart beats in a pregnant woman. External monitoring involves two external belts, one measuring uterine contractions and the other measuring the fetal heart rate. Internal monitoring requires ruptured membranes, after which an internal catheter is placed to measure uterine contractions, and an electrode is placed on the fetal scalp to measure the fetal heart beat directly. (See Appendix B.)

Morphine: a narcotic used for pain relief or for initial treatment of premature labor.

Myoma: a benign muscle overgrowth of the uterus (see fibroid).

Necrotizing enterocolitis (NEC): a bowel condition that may develop in a premature newborn, usually resulting from decreased blood flow to a portion of the intestine.

Nembutol: a barbiturate often used as a sleeping pill.

Neonatologist: a physician who is a pediatrician and who also has had an additional one or two years of training in neonatology (the care of the complicated newborn).

Nisentil: a short-acting narcotic often used in labor to take the "edge off contractions."

Nitrazine test: a test using litmus paper to determine whether or not the membranes have ruptured.

Os: opening (e.g., of cervix).

Patent ductus arteriosus: a heart condition in which a fetal blood vessel persists in the newborn, creating an abnormal flow of blood. This condition can resolve on its own, but may require medication or surgery.

Pediatrician: a physician who has completed three years of a pediatric residency specializing in the care of infants and children.

Pessary: a diaphragm-like ring that can be inserted into the vagina in order to further support the cervix and the uterus; commonly used to discourage any premature cervical effacement.

Placenta: the "afterbirth" that nourishes the unborn baby during pregnancy.

Placental abruption: a premature separation of the placenta from the wall of the uterus.

Placenta previa: implanting of the placenta over the internal cervical os, which prevents a vaginal delivery and often causes vaginal bleeding and premature labor. If a placenta previa persists at term, a Cesarean section is required for delivery.

Pneumonia: an infection of the lungs.

Polyhydramnios: excessive amniotic fluid in the uterus, which can contribute to development of premature labor.

Premature labor: the onset of uterine contractions causing cervical change prior to thirty-seven weeks of gestation. (See Preterm labor.)

Preterm labor: the onset of uterine contractions causing cervical change in a pregnancy that is less than thirty-seven weeks. (See Premature labor.)

PROM: a condition in which the membranes have ruptured but there is no onset of uterine contractions for twenty-four hours.

Pulse: number of heartbeats per minute. To measure your pulse: Place the index finger and third finger of your left hand on your inner right wrist, about half an inch from the bend of the wrist. Press gently and you will feel a soft throbbing. Count the number of these beats in a one-minute period.

Pyelonephritis: an infection of the kidneys.

Resident doctor: a physician who has completed medical school and is training in a specialty. The pediatric residency program has three levels: PL1, PL2, PL3, depending upon the year of training of the physician.

Respirator: a machine that assists breathing when the lungs are incapable of functioning on their own.

Respiratory distress syndrome (RDS): lung disease in a newborn caused by lung immaturity (hyaline membrane disease).

Ritodrine: a medication used in the treatment of premature labor.

Saddle block: spinal anesthesia placed in the spinal canal to numb the lower half of the body. (See Appendix B.)

Seconal: a barbiturate used as a sleeping aid.

Sepsis: a life-threatening infection that has invaded the bloodstream.

Sonogram: see ultrasound.

Spina bifida: a birth defect involving an opening of the spine in which there are exposed nerves without the usual bony protection (meningomyelocele).

Spinal anesthesia: anesthesia placed through a needle into the spinal canal, numbing the lower half of the body.

Terbutaline: a medication used in the treatment of premature labor.

Tocolytics: any medication that stops uterine contractions.

Trendelenburg: a position assumed when the hips are placed above shoulder level, e.g., a bed is tilted with the foot elevated at a five-degree angle in relationship to the shoulders.

Ultrasound: an examination of a part of the body using sound waves. A picture in gray and white shadows is created by the reflection of the sound waves. (See Appendix B.)

Umbilical cord catheter (UA line): a small catheter that is placed through the umbilical artery of the newborn baby in order to draw frequent samples of blood for various tests.

Vasodilan: a medication used for the treatment of premature labor.

Weakened cervix: a cervix that has prematurely dilated or effaced before the thirty-seventh week of gestation in the absence of any uterine contractions.

APPENDIX B

MEDICAL PROCEDURES

AMNIOCENTESIS

Amniocentesis is the withdrawal of amniotic fluid from around the fetus. When the amniocentesis is performed at four months of pregnancy, it is often done for genetic studies (e.g., evaluation for Down's syndrome) and for assessing the spinal cord of the fetus to rule out spina bifida. However, when the amniocentesis is performed in relationship to premature labor, it is done either to assess the maturity of the fetal lungs or to rule out any infection in the amniotic sac surrounding the fetus (chorioamnionitis). The amniocentesis is usually done in the hospital with the guidance of an ultrasound examination of the uterus, to determine the correct location for the placement of the needle in order to withdraw the amniotic fluid safely (avoiding the fetus, placenta, and umbilical cord).

Your partner can often be present during the amniocentesis, and you can both do shallow, slow breathing for relaxation (see Chapter Eight). The actual sensation of having an amniocentesis feels like a pinch, or like having blood drawn from a place other than the arm. Often a local injection of a numbing medication is given in the skin (e.g., similar to Novocaine at the dentist's); however, some physicians or patients prefer to use just one insertion of the needle without the local anesthesia.

Once the amniocentesis needle has been inserted into the uterus, about five teaspoons of the amniotic fluid are withdrawn (this fluid is replaced naturally by the fetus within two hours). After the fluid is withdrawn, the heart rate of the baby is monitored. It is important that you are on bedrest the next twenty-four hours after an amniocentesis so that no activity will interfere with the healing over of the hole in the membranes made by the amniocentesis needle.

The tests done on the amniotic fluid are then sent to the laboratory. If the amniocentesis has been done for the evaluation of the maturity of the fetal lungs, three different tests are usually performed that take approximately eight to ten hours to complete. The names of these tests are L/S ratio, PG, and PI. The initials represent different chemical tests, each in a different way determining the status of the fetal lungs. Often the results of these three tests together are grouped as follows: immature lungs, transitional lungs, and mature lungs. If the amniocentesis is done to check for infection, a microscopic exam of the fluid is done immediately (a Gram stain). If a number of bacteria are present, then an infection in the amniotic fluid is suspected. A culture of the fluid is also sent to the laboratory to determine if any bacteria will grow over the next few days.

Although theoretically the amniotic fluid that has been withdrawn could also be sent for genetic studies at the time of the amniocentesis, this is usually not done because of the extra expense (about $500) and the waiting period required for the results of the chromosomal analysis (three weeks).

The risks of amniocentesis may include premature leaking of amniotic fluid through the vagina (which usually resolves with bedrest), an increase in premature labor contractions (which may necessitate the use of medication to control them), fetal or placental bleeding (which usually resolves spontaneously), and the development of an infection around the baby (though this happens only on rare occasions; if it developed, the baby would need to be delivered immediately). Only occasionally has a "dimple" been reported in a baby who has undergone amniocentesis (possibly from the amniocentesis needle). Overall, the risks of an amniocentesis with ultrasound guidance are between 0.1 and 1 percent (very low, considering the importance of the information to be gained in the acute situation). Most women who have an amniocentesis do quite well.

ANESTHESIA

Ideally, there would be no need for anesthesia in any procedure done for labor and delivery. However, especially in a high-risk pregnancy, anesthesia is sometimes indicated for the medical safety of the mother and/or baby. Anesthesia is indicated in high-risk pregnancies in such cases as the placement of a cervical cerclage, the labor and impending delivery of a premature infant (e.g., epidural anesthesia to protect the soft head of the baby against the powerful forces of pushing), and the labor of a mother with high blood pressure (to keep the mother's blood pressure under control, thereby avoiding serious complications such as strokes and seizures).

There are a variety of anesthesia alternatives. They range from a simple injection of a narcotic such as Nisentil (used to take the "edge off" the labor contractions) to regional anesthesia (spinal or epidural) to general anesthesia (going to sleep).

Simple narcotics used in labor for pain relief include Nisentil and Demerol. Each of these medications lasts about one and a half to three hours, depending upon the dose. If the medication is given in labor, it must be timed appropriately; if it is given too close to the time of birth, it may affect the baby's initial respirations, slowing them down. However, the effect of the medication on the baby can be reversed with another medication called Narcan if the baby is born unexpectedly close to the time of the dose of the narcotic. If a narcotic medication is given too soon in labor (e.g., before the cervix is four cm dilated), it can slow labor down. It can also speed labor up, however, by helping the mother to relax between the contractions. The medication simply "takes the edge off" the contractions; the mother is still alert, and will need to use breathing techniques to tolerate the contractions.

A spinal or "saddle block" anesthetic can be used either as the baby is delivering, for a Cesarean section, or for a cerclage. Medication is placed through a small needle in the back into the spinal canal. This medication numbs the lower part of the body, usually lasting about two hours. One situation in which spinal anesthesia is used is the anticipated use of forceps. The forceps can be applied painlessly after a saddleblock is working, and the baby can be gently helped out of the vagina. A spinal is sometimes used for Cesarean sections, although some anesthesiologists prefer epidural anesthesia for this operation. A spinal is sometimes the anesthesia of choice for the placement of a cerclage, as only a small amount of medication used, thereby reducing risk that any of it might cross over to the baby (the baby is usually at sixteen to twenty-eight weeks of gestation at the time of the cerclage).

Spinal anesthesia is placed while the mother is either sitting up or lying on her side, curled up in the "fetal position" with her back pushed out "like a cat." This position is critical for the proper placement of the spinal, as it is more difficult to find the right space between the bones of the back when one is pregnant and has extra weight. A very small needle is used, to minimize the risk of headaches (which occur in about 1 percent of patients receiving spinal anesthesia; the headache can be corrected with oral or IV fluids to the mother, or by a procedure called a "blood patch"). Once the spinal anesthesia has been placed, it is important that the mother lie flat in bed for twelve to twenty-four hours to allow the small hole in the spinal canal (created by the spinal needle) to heal over (a spinal headache may be caused by the leaking of spinal fluid from this hole).

Epidural anesthesia is a regional anesthesia that also numbs the lower body. However, the medication is injected in the back, not directly into the spinal canal, but into the epidural space, which is next to the spinal canal. An epidural anesthetic takes longer, and is technically more difficult to place than a spinal (not all anesthesiologists do epidurals routinely). The advantages of an epidural are that little medication, if any, crosses over to the baby, and there is less risk of a "spinal" headache, as the medication does not go directly into the spinal canal. An epidural is placed in the same manner as a spinal anesthetic, in terms of the mother's position. An epidural can be used in labor to numb the uterus from the pain of the contractions. Often a small catheter is placed in the epidural space with the initial epidural medication so that the medication can be reinjected at regular intervals as needed during labor. An epidural is often used for a Cesarean section. Because of the low risk for headache, the mother has no restrictions on her position following the Cesarean after epidural anesthesia (which comes in handy when breastfeeding).

General anesthesia is rarely used; however, in certain situations it is necessary.

For instance, if a fetus gets into trouble during labor, there is often not time to place either an epidural or a spinal block for anesthesia (ten to twenty minutes). The baby needs to be delivered immediately, so general anesthesia is used. For a baby in distress, general anesthesia is also safer, as it provides a better environment if the acid-base balance of the baby is disturbed as a result of stress. It is sometimes scary to have general anesthesia for a Cesarean section, as you would usually prefer to be awake for the birth. However, no matter how chaotic the situation, if unexpected distress occurs and there is need for a Cesarean section with general anesthesia, remember that the best thing for the baby is being done, and that general anesthesia is usually quite safe. Often a mask with oxygen is placed on your face first, and then Pentothal is injected into an IV. Once the Pentothal takes effect (one to two minutes) and you are asleep, a tube is inserted into your airway and the operation begins as additional gases are given through the tube. The baby is usually delivered quickly (five to ten minutes from the time the Cesarean section begins) to minimize any transfer of the anesthesia gases to the baby. The gases used for the anesthesia are "light" gases, and usually you are alert within a half an hour from the end of the Cesarean section, and are able to breastfeed at that time. It is thought, since only colostrum is present at this time directly after the birth, and the actual milk "comes in" on the third day, that little if any of the anesthesia gas is passed to the baby during this first breastfeeding. It is very important to get the baby used to the nipple of the breast and begin the stimulation of sucking so that milk will "come in" on time. However, occasionally after a Cesarean section with the mother under general anesthesia, the baby is a little "sleepy" for twelve to twenty-four hours and may not nurse well. If this happens, do not worry. However, if the baby does not nurse well after this twenty-four-hour period, it is important to begin using the electric breast pump and to ask for additional nursing instruction.

After any operation, medications are often used for the comfort of the mother, and antibiotics may be needed to prevent or treat an infection. Your obstetrician is familiar with these medications, keeping in mind that they may cross the placenta or breast milk. If you need these medications, e.g., for pain, nausea, or sleep, do not hold back from using them.

In conclusion, although both mothers and obstetricians would prefer that no anesthesia be given during pregnancy or at the time of the birth, occasionally it is necessary. Nowadays spinal, epidural, and general anesthesia are all relatively safe. If you are undergoing anesthesia, talk it over with your anesthesiologist in detail, relating your individual medical history. Between the three of you (yourself, your obstetrician, and your anesthesiologist), a decision will be made as to which type of anesthesia is best in your situation.

CULTURES

Cultures are tests done to check for a viral (e.g., herpes) or bacterial (e.g., strep) infection. These infections can occur in various parts of the body. In pregnancy, infections that are often evaluated include those of the vagina (vaginitis), bladder (lower urinary tract infection or cystitis), kidney (upper urinary tract infection or pyelonephritis), and pregnant uterus (chorioamnionitis). The infections may be either the cause or the result of the preterm labor, and it is very important to check for them thoroughly.

Sometimes, if the infection is severe, there are obvious symptoms, e.g., fever. However, occasionally in pregnancy an infection may be present although the symptoms are subtle (e.g., increased frequency of urination that is indistinguishable from the normally increased urination in pregnancy), or there may be no symptoms at all. Thus, testing is very important to determine the presence of an infection. A culture of the suspect area is taken and if it is positive, the infection is definitely present. However, occasionally the culture may be negative, but the symptoms are still present and another test may indicate or suggest that there is an infection. For instance, if a pregnant woman has symptoms of a bladder infection and although a culture may be negative, a microscopic examination reveals inflammatory cells, the infection may very well be present and may respond to antibiotics.

A culture usually takes forty-eight to seventy-two hours to grow out any bacteria on the culture plate. More specialized cultures, e.g., herpes cultures, might take two weeks for a final interpretation. If the culture is for abnormal bacteria, and the bacteria do grow out, the bacteria are then typed (given a name) and antibiotic sensitivities are evaluated. In some instances, some bacteria may be resistant to a particular antibiotic, such as penicillin, but sensitive to another antibiotic, such as Keflex. Usually these sensitivities evaluated in the laboratory reflect those of the bacteria in the body of the pregnant woman at that time to a specific antibiotic.

Once an infection has been diagnosed and treated, it is usually important to reevaluate the site of infection for a possible recurrence of infection. Therefore, if a woman has had a bladder infection that has been treated with an antibiotic, once the course of antibiotics is completed it is very important to have another urine sample taken for a culture to be sure the bladder infection has cleared.

Urine Cultures

The bladder and kidneys are frequent sites of infection during pregnancy. Normally the urine should contain no bacteria (it should be sterile). Reliable cultures of the urine are obtained by the midstream method (separating the labial folds of the vagina, placing a small amount of urine in the toilet, and catching the rest in midstream with a sterile container). The reason for this method is that there are normally bacteria in the vagina, and often the initial part of the urine stream does carry some vaginal bacteria with it. By catching the "midstream" sample of urine, the possibility of "contamination" of vaginal bacteria in the urine is minimized.

A urine culture takes approximately twenty-four to forty-eight hours for interpretation. Previously, the definition of a positive bladder infection was based on the presence of 100,000 bacterial colonies per culture plate inoculated with urine. However, we now know that in women, especially in those with premature labor, a bacterial count of even 10,000 of one type of bacteria may be significant. Antibiotic sensitivities are usually run on the bacteria that may be grown in the culture plate.

Vaginal Cultures

The vagina is normally the home of many different bacteria. However, occasionally there are bacteria that can cause an infection (1) by having one normal population of bacteria in the vagina overgrow and dominate the other populations, or (2) by the introduction of foreign bacteria. The vaginal culture is usually ready for evaluation at forty-eight hours after inoculation with a culture swab from the vaginal secretions. Some bacteria that grow out from the vaginal culture are normal bacteria in the vagina, such as "lactobacillus"; however, others may be definitely abnormal, such as gonorrhea. Sometimes an overgrowth of yeast is present that can be safely treated in pregnancy with a local cream.

For pregnant patients, there is a particular type of bacteria of significance that 5 percent of women normally carry in the vagina: Group B Strep. If a pregnant woman has Group B Strep present in the vagina and goes on to have a premature delivery, the baby is at risk (having been exposed to the Group B Strep in the vaginal canal) for developing a life-threatening infection. Therefore, a woman in premature labor is usually evaluated for the presence of Group B Strep in her vagina, and if it is present, antibiotics are often prescribed. Although this is not a venereal disease, the Group B Strep bacteria can be passed back and forth between the pregnant woman and her partner with subsequent intercourse; therefore it is important for her partner also to take the antibiotics at the same time.

Amniotic Fluid Cultures

A culture of amniotic fluid (withdrawn at the time of amniocentesis) is sometimes done, to rule out any infection around the fetus. This culture is evaluated at both twenty-four and forty-eight hours. Normally the amniotic fluid around the fetus is sterile, and there should be no growth of any bacteria. If there is some bacterial growth, the possibility of chorioamnionitis needs to be seriously considered, depending upon the clinical situation of the pregnant woman. Immediate delivery of the fetus is indicated if a diagnosis of clinical Chorioamnionitis is made. Chorioamnionitis (an infection around the fetus) is life-threatening for the baby.

Because such an infection can be very serious, and because the culture can take one to two days for evaluation, a Gram strain is often performed immediately from the amniotic fluid. This is done by placing a drop of amniotic fluid on a glass slide and evaluating the slide microscopically. There should be no bacteria on the slide. Occasionally there can be an inflammatory cell, which is of little significance. The result of this test is then evaluated, together with the overall clinical situation at the time.

INTRAVENOUS FLUIDS

Occasionally, intravenous (IV) fluids are required during the treatment of premature labor, either for the administration of fluids for hydration, or for medication to stop the premature labor contractions. The IV is a small, flexible catheter inserted via a needle into the vein of your hand or your arm. It is then attached by tubing to a bag or bottle of balanced salt solution. These solutions provide a minimal amount of calories. Sometimes the insertion of the needle may be slightly uncomfortable, and it can be helpful to do the relaxation exercises found in Chapter Eight.

Once the IV is inserted, the Teflon catheter and tubing are securely taped in place and any discomfort usually subsides over the next few hours. Both the tubing and the catheter will move with you as your position changes. Be protective of them, but do not let them restrict your movements. Just be sure the IV does not get tangled or compressed. The IV catheter will be changed every forty-eight hours to avoid any inflammation of the vein by the catheter—if, in fact, the IV needs to stay in the vein that long.

MONITORING

Two types of monitoring are used in obstetrics: external and internal. In evaluating a pregnant woman for possible premature labor, external monitoring *only* is used. Two belts are placed around the pregnant abdomen. The first belt, or "toco," is used for the detection of uterine contractions. A simple pressure gauge presses against the external skin on the top of the pregnant uterus. When a contraction or tightening occurs, a signal is transmitted via the cord on the belt to the machine, and a printout in the machine records the contraction. Recently, a home monitor has been developed to help pregnant women with preterm labor detect the contractions more accurately. Currently, these monitors are only experimental.

Early preterm labor contractions are often not painful. Many pregnant women are barely aware of them. For some women, they feel like cramps or mild pressure. Often they are confused with gas or fetal movement. The external monitor will confirm the existence of the uterine contractions and can often help you to identify them. Occasionally you may feel a contraction and note that it is not registering on the monitor. If that is the case, notify the nurse who is taking care of you, as the monitor or your belt may need to be adjusted (in preterm labor, it is important that the belt monitoring the uterine contractions be below the naval). The external uterine belt measures the frequency of the contractions but not their strength.

Sometimes irritability of the uterus is present but not actual contractions. Uterine irritability registers in little waves, with the potential of uterine contractions breaking out every so often.

If no contractions or irritability are present, the monitor should register a fairly flat line, only occasionally interrupted by such normal events as fetal movement, laughing, or turning in the bed.

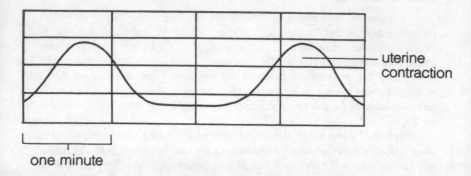

Figure 7. Monitor strip showing uterine contractions.

The second belt placed around the abdomen is to detect the fetal heartbeat. This part of the external monitor uses an ultrasound sensor to pick up the fetal heart. Early in pregnancy especially, the fetus is very active and difficult to record continuously. Therefore, often the heartbeat is counted for a few minutes and then the external belt for the fetus is discontinued.

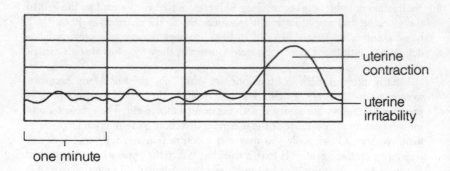

Figure 8. Monitor strip showing uterine irritability with occasional contractions.

The normal heartbeat of the fetus varies between 110 to 160 beats per minute. It may fluctuate on the external monitor tracing, and in fact this is desirable, as more variability indicates a healthier fetal nervous system. If all of a sudden the

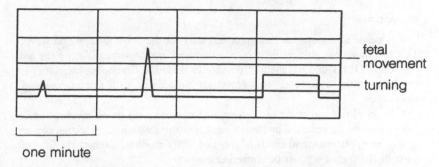

Figure 9. Monitor strip with no evidence of preterm labor.

heartbeat goes from 160 to 0, do not panic. It usually only means that the baby has moved out of the range of the ultrasound sensor, and the belt simply needs to be readjusted in order to re-locate the fetal heartbeat.

Even though you may have one or two external belts on for an extended period of time, do not let them restrict your movements from side to side in bed, as this position change is important. It is also important to have the nurse change the belts' positions on a regular basis, so that skin irritation does not occur.

Internal monitoring is used only if the membranes around the baby are ruptured and delivery is anticipated in a few hours. Again, there are two parts to the internal monitor. The first part measures the uterine contractions. A small catheter is inserted into the uterus under sterile conditions to measure the frequency and strength of the uterine contractions. The second part is the internal fetal monitor. A small clip is placed on the baby's scalp to directly measure the heartbeat of the baby with an electrical signal. Internal monitoring is usually reserved for special situations, e.g., suspicion that the baby is having trouble tolerating labor, or abnormal slowing of progress in labor.

The fetal monitor is a valuable diagnostic tool, but remember that it is only a machine. The information it provides is only one aspect of the total picture. Sometimes it may seem that the doctors and nurses are more interested in the monitor than in you. Some couples fall into the habit of watching the monitor printout more avidly than they would watch a good movie. Avoid the pitfall of letting the monitor totally dominate your thoughts and feelings; this will only increase your feelings of isolation and anxiety. Make the monitor your tool, not vice versa. Many women find it reassuring to have the monitor on. It means you do not always have to be alert to the next contraction: you can relax and let the monitor pick it up. Using the monitor can also be an opportunity to use some relaxation techniques during contractions (see Chapters Two and Eight).

ULTRASOUND

A pelvic ultrasound, or sonogram, is a study of the pelvis using sound waves. This technique has only recently been introduced into obstetrics (during the last ten years). Ultrasound has made it possible to study the developing pregnancy in depth, and also to perform some obstetrical procedures, such as amniocentesis, more safely.

In an ultrasound study of the pregnant uterus, sound waves are directed to the uterus and are reflected by the different structures within it, creating a picture of the fetus, placenta, and cervix in gray and white shadows. Each of the integral parts of the pregnancy can be studied extensively.

The fetus (or fetuses—the ultrasound will determine if there are more than one) can be studied in many different parameters. An estimate of the biparietal diameter (BPD) is usually made, when the position of the fetus permits it. This measurement (in centimeters) measures the distance between two points on the fetal skull, and can give a fairly accurate estimation of the number of weeks of gestation (plus or minus two weeks), thereby confirming the due date or establishing a new one. However, this accuracy can vary, depending upon the week of gestation during which the ultrasound is done. The most accurate estimation of the due date according to the biparietal diameter is made when the gestational age is between fifteen and twenty-five weeks.

The different parts of the fetal body can also be studied: the arms, legs, bladder, kidneys, spinal cord, and heart chambers. The abdominal circumference is measured to rule out delayed fetal growth, along with a measurement of the length of the femur (thigh bone). Some birth defects can be diagnosed, e.g., spina

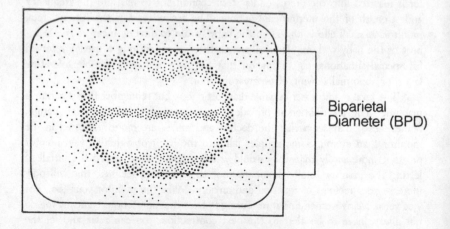

Biparietal
Diameter (BPD)

Figure 10. Ultrasound measurement of the fetal head diameter.

bifida or "opening of the spinal canal." Some conditions, such as Down's syndrome, cannot be detected by ultrasound.

The placenta can be examined for signs of early maturation, and also for its location in the uterus. If the placenta has implanted over the internal cervical os, creating a placenta previa, this can usually be seen with the ultrasound. If the placenta has separated prematurely from the wall of the uterus (placental abruption), this can often also be seen on the ultrasound if greater than a 30 percent to 50 percent area of the placenta has been involved in the separation.

The amount of amniotic fluid is also evaluated. Too much amniotic fluid can contribute to premature labor, or indicate the presence of diabetes in the pregnant woman. Too little amniotic fluid may indicate a poorly functioning fetal bladder, or may be the first sign of a possible slowing down of fetal growth.

Sometimes the ultrasound can detect abnormalities of the uterus, such as uterine myomas or fibroids (benign tumors of the uterus that may grow rapidly as a result of the pregnancy hormones and may also contribute to premature labor).

The risks to humans of an ultrasound examination have not yet been studied on a long-term basis. However, ultrasound has been used for about ten years in obstetrics and so far no harmful effects have been documented in the children, now ten years old, who were exposed in utero. Because some questions have been raised about the safety of ultrasound to the fetus, it is not recommended that ultrasound be routinely used in every normal pregnancy until more is known about its long-term effects. The questions of safety revolve around the amount of heat to which the fetal cells are exposed during the ultrasound examination. Obviously there is more worry early in pregnancy, when the fetus is quite small, than in later pregnancy, where there are more fetal cells and more diffusion of the same amount of ultrasound during the time period of the study. As always in a complex situation, the possible risks of the ultrasound must be weighed against the potential benefits.

For the premature labor patient, a baseline ultrasound is often obtained for several reasons, including reaffirmation of the due date in order to properly treat the premature labor; the screening out of any possible contributing causes to the premature labor, such as the presence of twins; excessive amniotic fluid; determination of placental location to rule out a placenta previa; evaluation of the placenta to rule out a placental abruption; evaluation of the fetus for any obvious birth defects; and establishment of a fetal growth curve in order to rule out any growth delay of the fetus.

VAGINAL EXAMINATION

The vaginal examination is an essential part of the evaluation for premature labor. However, if there is any significant amount of vaginal bleeding, an ultrasound usually precedes the examination to rule out a placenta previa. (If a vaginal exam is done and a placenta previa is present, a hemorrhage may ensue. Therefore, if there is any significant vaginal bleeding present, the exam is postponed.)

The vaginal examination is usually done in two parts. If there is any suspicion of ruptured membranes, a "sterile speculum" examination is done. A sterile speculum is inserted into the vagina while you are lying in bed (sometimes with your bottom propped upon a bedpan), and several samples of vaginal secretions are withdrawn. Two tests are often done immediately on the vaginal secretion samples. The first is a Nitrazine test, in which litmus paper turns blue (initially yellow) if there has been any leaking of amniotic fluid. However, if there has been recent intercourse, this test can be positive even though there may be no leaking of the amniotic fluid. The second test is a "fern test," in which a sample of vaginal fluid is examined under the microscope for a pattern of ferns, indicating leakage of amniotic fluid. If there are several teaspoons of fluid in the vagina, a sample may be obtained to be sent to the laboratory to determine fetal lung maturity (PG test). A culture is also often taken from the vagina to check for any vaginal infection.

The second part of the vaginal examination is the palpation (feeling) of the cervix in the vagina. It is important to evaluate the dilation, effacement, consistency, and axis of the cervix in the vagina, and the position of the baby in the pelvis. This part of the exam is usually repeated at certain intervals, as long as the membranes are not ruptured. Sometimes vaginal examinations can be uncomfortable. Try the slow breathing described in Chapter Eight to help you relax. If you can relax during the examination, the examiner can be more accurate in the assessment of the cervix and the position of the fetus, and you will be more comfortable. If the membranes are ruptured, however, this part of the examination is usually omitted, so that the risk of infection from the vaginal bacteria ascending up the birth canal to the baby is not increased.

BIBLIOGRAPHY

FETAL DEVELOPMENT

Nilsson, Lennart. *A Child Is Born: The Drama of Life before Birth*, Rev., 1977.

Rugh, Robert and Landrum Shettles. *From Conception to Birth: The Drama of Life's Beginnings*, 1971.

Verney, Thomas and Kelly John. *Secret Life of the Unborn Child*, 1981.

PREGNANCY

Brown, Judith. *Nutrition for Your Pregnancy*, 1984.

Bing, Elizabeth. *Making Love During Pregnancy*, 1982.

Elkins, Valani. *The Rights of the Pregnant Parent*, 1980.

Kitzinger, Sheila. *The Complete Book of Childbirth and Pregnancy*, 1980.

McCauley, Carole. *Pregnancy After Thirty-five*, 1978.

Wilson, Christine and Wendy Hovey. *Cesarean Childbirth: A Handbook for Parents*, 1980.

HIGH-RISK PREGNANCY (PRETERM LABOR, PREMATURE BABIES, ETC.)

Freeman, Roger and Pescar. *Safe Delivery: Protecting Your Baby During High Risk Pregnancy*, 1982.

Hales, Dianne, and Robert Creasy. *New Hope for Problem Pregnancies*, 1982.

Harrison, Helen. *The Premature Baby Book; Parents' Guide to Coping and Caring in the First Year*, 1983.

Nance, Sherri. *Premature Babies: A Handbook for Parents*, 1982.

PREGNANCY LOSS

Friedman, Rochelle, and Bonnie Gradstein. *Surviving Pregnancy Loss*, 1982.

Scweibert, Pat, and Paul Kirk. *When Hello Means Good-bye*, 1981.

CHILDBIRTH EDUCATION

Bing, Elizabeth. *Six Practical Lessons for an Easier Childbirth*, 1977.

BOOKS FOR CHILDREN

Alexander, Martha. *When the New Baby Comes, I Am Moving Out*, 1979. (Encourages expression of feelings of resentment.)

Banish, Roslyn. *I Want to Tell You About My Baby*, 1982. (Photos and clear text describe emotions and present information about pregnancy and babies.)

Brooks, Robert. *So That's How I Was Born*, 1983. (Illustrated presentation of conception and birth.)

Cole, Joanna. *How You Were Born*, 1984. (Photographs accompanied by simple text for children, explaining fetal development, birth, and the experience of being a sibling.)

Hoban, Russell. *A Baby Sister for Frances*, 1964. (A story about a little badger that enacts many children's probable ambivalence about the upcoming birth.)

BREASTFEEDING

Eiger, Marvin and Sally Wendkos Olds. *The Complete Book of Breast Feeding*, 1972.

Prior, Karen. *Nursing Your Baby*, 1973.

INFANT CARE

Leach, Penelope. *Your Baby and Child*, 1977.

Spock, Benjamin. *Baby and Child Care*, 1976.

CHILD DEVELOPMENT/PARENTING

Brazelton, T. Berry. *Infants and Mothers: Differences in Development*, 1969.

Brazelton, T. Berry. *On Becoming a Family: The Growth of Attachment*, 1981.

Dally, Ann. *Inventing Motherhood: The Consequences of an Ideal*, 1983.

Dodson, Fitzhugh. *How to Parent*, 1970.

Gaffe, Viertel. *Becoming Parents: Preparing for the Emotional Changes of First Time Parenthood*, 1979.

Princeton Center for Infancy and Early Education. *The First Twelve Months*, 1973.

CHILD CARE

Bodin, Jeanne and Bonnie Mitelman. *Mothers Who Work: Strategies for Coping,*
  1983.
Siegel-Gorelick, Bryna. *The Working Parents' Guide to Child Care: How to Find
  the Best Care for Your Child,* 1983.

INDEX

Note: Italicized page numbers refer to illustrations.

C

anxiety and, 61–62
changes in sexual relations and, 52–55
coping with, 61–62, 65–67
in family members, 69
family members' assistance in dealing with, 86–88
feelings of powerlessness and, 44–47
financial changes and, 42–44
life role changes and, 36–42
loss of with fantasized pregnancy, 55–57
origins of, 59
outlets for, 59–60
premature labor caused by, 32
relaxation exercises for, 62–64
worksheet for, 61, 65–67
worries about the baby and, 29–36
Sugar, 154–55
Support networks, 80–82
Sutures. *See* Cerclages
Swimming, 160

T

Tao Te Ching, 176
Telephones: mobile, 107
Television watching, 106
Terbutaline, 14, 190
Time pressures, 102–3
antidotes for, 103–5
Tocolytics, 13, 190
Trendelenburg position, 5, 11, *12*, 23, 160, 190
Twins, 8

U

UA line. *See* Umbilical artery catheters
Ultrasound measurements, 4, 10, 23, 190, *202*, 202–3
Ulven, Mary Sue, 110, 144
Umbilical artery catheters (UA line), 130, 191
Unproductivity: feelings of, 37–38
Urine cultures, 197–98
Uterine irritability, 199, *200*
Uterus
anatomy of, 3, *4*
muscle strength in, 125–26

V

Vaginal cultures, 198
Vaginal examinations, 113, 203–4
Varicose veins, 13
Vasodilan, 14, 191
Visualization
academic and business uses of, 169–70
changes resulting from, 170–71
dictation for, 173
exercises
Creating Stillness, 175–76
The Healing Stream, 174–75
Inner Physician, 178
The Meadow, 174
Special Place, 176–78
history of, 169
images experienced during, 172

218   *Index*

involvement of partners in, 95,
    173, 174, 175
medical uses of, 170
personal story re, 170–71
process of, 171–72, 173
return to waking state and, 173

W

Waldholz-Goldblatt, Elysa, 20–21
Weakened cervix. *See* Cervix,
    weakened
Worries about the baby
re baby's health, 29, 35
coping with, 30, 33–34
feelings of ambivalence about,
    31–32
guilt feelings and, 32–33
imaginings of past loss and, 30
partners' worries, 30–31
preoccupation with bodily
    details and, 30
psychological consultation for,
    31
self-examination of attitudes
    and, 32
talking with others about, 33
use of denial for, 31

Z

Zukor, Joan and Lee, 91

**Cassette Tape on Prenatal Exercises
for the Pregnant Woman on Bedrest
by Femmy De Lyser, R.N.,
and Patricia Robertson, M.D.**

This thirty-minute cassette tape guides the pregnant woman on bedrest through prenatal exercises designed specifically for her, so that she may maintain her muscle tone and be more comfortable despite her confinement to bed. Accompanying the tape is a letter to your obstetrician discussing the exercises, and their implication for your specific situation.

For your copy of the tape, please send $8.95 (check or money order) to:

*Women's Medical Research Foundation
700 Arizona Avenue
Santa Monica, CA 90401*

"Hypnosis for Pregnancy"
a cassette tape by
Jan Berlin, Ph.D.

This sixty-minute cassette tape offers practical steps for the use of hypnosis during pregnancy.

Side One: Self-Hypnosis for Couples in Premature Labor *emphasizes positive self-talk and the use of hypnosis for creating relaxation, as well as for revitalization and energy. Specific suggestions are designed for both members of the couple in premature labor. Couples may use the tape to reaffirm the presence of both inner and outer resources which can help them to sustain their pregnancy.*

Side Two: Applications of Hypnosis for Childbirth *includes hypnotic techniques specifically designed to increase comfort and provide couples with a greater sense of control during labor. Tailored to work with child-birth education methods, the tape teaches partners how to give suggestions, including posthypnotic suggestions, and emphasizes deepening the couple's alliance during labor.*

Jan Berlin, Ph.D., is a licensed clinical psychologist and a past member of the visiting faculty at UCLA. Specializing in the use of clinical hypnosis and visualization techniques, he has worked with artists, athletes, students, and corporate managers to promote creativity and excellence. Dr. Berlin has helped couples in premature labor to recognize their own resourcefulness in sustaining their pregnancies.

To receive a copy of the tape, send your request to MAXXIS, Inc., 619 S. Vulcan Avenue, Suite 204, Encinitas, CA 92024. Please include a check or money order for $10 with your request (includes shipping and handling).